Margaret Humphreys

Plague and Fire

PLAGUE and FIRE

*Battling Black Death and the
1900 Burning of Honolulu's Chinatown*

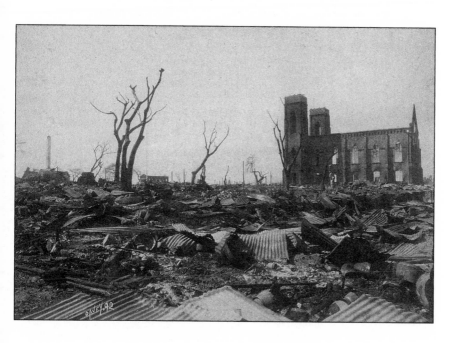

James C. Mohr

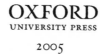

OXFORD
UNIVERSITY PRESS

2005

OXFORD
UNIVERSITY PRESS

Oxford   New York
Auckland   Bangkok   Buenos Aires   Cape Town   Chennai
Dar es Salaam   Delhi   Hong Kong   Istanbul   Karachi   Kolkata
Kuala Lumpur   Madrid   Melbourne   Mexico City   Mumbai   Nairobi
São Paulo   Shanghai   Taipei   Tokyo   Toronto

Copyright © 2005 by Oxford University Press, Inc.

Published by Oxford University Press, Inc.
198 Madison Avenue, New York, New York 10016
www.oup.com

Oxford is a registered trademark of Oxford University Press

Library of Congress Cataloging-in-Publication Data
Mohr, James C.
Plague and fire: battling black death and the burning of
Honolulu's Chinatown / James C. Mohr.
p. cm. Includes bibliographical references and index.
ISBN 0-19-516231-5
1. Plague—Hawaii—Honolulu—History—19th century.
2. Chinatown (Honolulu, Hawaii)—History—19th century.
3. Fires—Hawaii—Honolulu—History—19th century.
I. Title
RC176.H3M64 2005
614.5'732'0996931—dc22   2004049223

1 3 5 7 9 8 6 4 2

Printed in the United States of America
on acid-free paper

For Elizabeth

Contents

Contents

Acknowledgments

This book had its origins over twenty years ago, when I was invited to lecture at the University of Hawaii. During my visit, I took a walk through the Chinatown district of Honolulu and happened to notice a modest sign on the front of a building. The sign informed passersby that none of the structures they were looking at were original because all of the original buildings in the area had been destroyed around 1900 in a fire ordered by the Board of Health. Perhaps because I was working at the time on a history of medical jurisprudence in the United States during the nineteenth century, and especially since I was in Hawaii to lecture on the intersection of medical and social policies, the sign instantly piqued my curiosity. Was the information correct? If so, why had local health officers implemented such a dramatic policy, and how had they acquired the power to do so? How did the city respond, and what happened to the people affected? To answer those and related questions, I began to collect material about the event, even as I finished other projects.

The sign itself disappeared shortly after I saw it, but I will always be grateful to whoever put it up.[1] It alerted me to an event I have found absolutely riveting for a host of reasons: it took place against the background of a worldwide epidemic of bubonic plague and involved physicians from different cultures caught in the middle of an unfinished revolution in public health practice; it took place in one of the most multicultural, multilingual, and multiethnic cities on the globe at the time and involved tense interracial dynamics; it took place in a context of political maneuvering that delivered the Kingdom of Hawaii to the United States and involved imperial visions that would put the archipelago on a path toward American statehood.

In my extended search for information about the Chinatown fire, I have benefited from the generous guidance of a great many people and the shared resources of a great many institutions. Historians simply cannot work without first-rate librarians and well-tended collections. In Honolulu, I am enormously indebted to Judith Kearney, Laura Gerwitz, and the staff of the Mamiya Medical Heritage Center and Historical Archive of the Hawaiian Medical Library. Their superb collection of physician files were invaluable for this research, and I am also grateful for their permission to use many of the physician portraits that appear in this book. I also want to thank Geoff White and the staff of the Hawaiian State Archives, where many of the key documents related to these events have been saved. The state archives likewise permitted the reproduction of illustrations.

Elsewhere in Honolulu, DeSoto Brown, Linda Laurence, and Judith Kearney (after she transferred there) were a pleasure to work with at the Bishop Museum Archives, as were Patty Lei and the staff of the Bishop Museum Library. James Ho of the Hawaiian Chinese Multicultural Museum provided wonderful insights and articles from his vast store of personal lore. Joan Hori, Susie Cheng, and the Special Collections staffs at Hamilton Library, University of Hawaii at Manoa, repeatedly helped me find materials and arranged special access where necessary. I would also like to acknowledge the help I received while using the collections of the Hawaiian State Library, the Hawaiian Historical Society, and the Hawaiian Mission Children's Society Library.

As in the past, working in the Historical Division of the National Library of Medicine in Bethesda, Maryland, proved both enjoyable and valuable. The staff of Archives II in Adelphi, Maryland, guided me through the papers of the United States Public Health Service, and John Parascandola, Historian of the Public Health Service, kindly offered access to records then stored in his office. Brooke Black at the Huntington Library in San Marino, California, helped me with the Nathaniel B. Emerson Papers, and the Buffalo and Erie County Historical Society Archives sent me material from the Francis L. Folsom Papers.

The more I learned about Honolulu's crisis of plague and fire, the more I wanted to find as many accounts as I could from people who experienced it. Moreover, I hoped to hear their stories as they were recorded for one another in their own languages, in memoirs and newspapers. Thanks to generous scholars who know Hawaiian, Chinese, and Japanese, I was able to do that. For translation from Hawaiian, I am greatly indebted to Richard Keao K. NeSmith. Then an instructor in Polynesian languages at the University of Hawaii at Manoa, NeSmith answered a plea for help from a scholar he had never met. Both his marvelous translations and the generosity of his academic spirit command my deepest admiration and respect. For translations from Chinese, I thank Yuhuan Li at the University of Hawaii, Manoa, and Jingzhu Wu at the University of Oregon. For translations from Japanese I thank Atsuko Fukunaga and Reiko Sawyer at the University of Hawaii, Manoa, and Eric Cunningham at the University of Oregon. My colleagues Arif Dirlik, Andrew Goble, Bryna Goodman, Jeff Hanes, and Ka-Che Yip were also wonderfully patient with many ad hoc questions related to Asian languages.

At the University of Oregon, I am fortunate to enjoy the outstanding services of the Knight Library, particularly the Interlibrary Loan division under Joanne Halgren and the Government Documents and Maps division under Tom Stave. Sheerin Shahinpoor was an outstanding research assistant. I also received the benefit of extremely useful feedback when I presented preliminary ideas and various portions of this material to several different groups. Among them were the International Congress for the History of Medicine, Tunis, 1998; the Pacific Coast Branch of the American Historical Association, Honolulu, 1999 (where I particularly want to thank David Chappell and Charles McClain); the Policy History Conference, St. Louis, 2002 (where I particularly want to thank Daniel Fox); the New York Academy of Medicine, 2002 (where I particularly want to thank Gerald Oppenheimer, Edward Morman, and the Galdston Lecture committee); and the International Congress for the History of Medicine, Istanbul, 2002.

Guenter Risse, the leading expert on this same plague in San Francisco, has shared his knowledge generously and appeared on academic panels with me. William Rothstein read my early essays on this subject and offered insightful comments. Arif Dirlik and Jeff Ostler both read the entire manuscript, for which I am most appreciative. I was extremely fortunate to work with Susan Ferber at Oxford University Press. Her excellent suggestions and editorial skills have made this book far better than it would otherwise have been. I also want to extend special thanks to Robert E. McGlone at the University of Hawaii, Manoa, who had originally invited me to speak in Honolulu and has continued to help advance this project in countless ways over many years.

Finally, my most enduring and profound sources of support continue to spring—as they have for almost four decades—from my wife, Betty, to whom this book is dedicated.

Plague and Fire

Prologue

Saturday, January 20, 1900, began as a soft and balmy morning, the kind of day that made Honolulu seem idyllic to people who remembered January in Chicago or New England. Under clear skies, the air temperature was climbing slowly through the low 70s. A light breeze wafted gently in from the ocean before turning up the steep slopes of the volcanic ridge, or *pali*, that rose behind the city. But three of the people out early that morning were not in the streets to enjoy the benign weather, even though two of them had grown up in Chicago and the third had spent several years in New England. Nathaniel B. Emerson, Francis R. Day, and Clifford B. Wood were physicians, and together they ran the Republic of Hawaii's Board of Health. For more than a month they had been directing a largely unsuccessful battle against the first invasion of bubonic plague ever to reach the Hawaiian islands.

Each morning the three physicians fanned out to visit already ailing patients, examine anyone newly reported sick, and inspect for themselves any sites around the city reported to be dangerous or unhealthful. The doctors then convened every day in a drab government office across from Honolulu's ornate Iolani Palace to review overnight developments, discuss their general policies, listen to the ideas or complaints of others, make decisions about what to do or try next, and issue the appropriate orders.

At 10:30 on this particular morning, the three doctors returned to their office, where they were joined by a civilian member of the Board of Health. Wood, who had taken over as Board president only two weeks before, formally called the group to order.

Although the civilian government of Hawaii had ceded absolute authority to the Board of Health during the plague emergency, the three physicians had so far been unable to halt the epidemic. They had imposed a military quarantine around the Chinatown district of Honolulu, where the bubonic plague had initially appeared and where all of the dead through mid-January had contracted the disease; they had spent hundreds of thousands of dollars from the Hawaiian treasury, mostly on clean-up efforts inside the quarantined zone; and for the last three weeks they had even been issuing orders to the fire department to burn buildings where plague victims had lived or worked. Regardless of what the doctors did, however, the epidemic was continuing to kill Chinatown residents at a steady rate of one or two every day. Even worse, the disease was spreading. A white woman in a prosperous neighborhood north of Chinatown had died just a few days earlier, and her death became front-page news in all of Honolulu's daily papers, including those published in Chinese, Japanese, and Hawaiian. The doctors feared the entire city was on the brink of a general panic.

To inhibit further spread of the disease in the week ahead, the three physicians began their meeting by passing an edict prohibiting all indoor assemblies throughout the city, including the following day's church services, until further notice. They next applied to the new plague site outside Chinatown the same policy they had already been implementing inside Chinatown: they ordered the fire department to add the home of the dead white woman to their ongoing list of buildings to burn. Shortly after 11:00 A.M., the Board members resumed a previously deferred discussion of other possible plague sites inside Chinatown. Earlier in the week they had ordered the burning of a cluster of shacks where two plague victims had been found dead. Those ramshackle wooden structures were located in what the doctors' quarantine map labeled as block 15, a compact rectangle that also housed Kaumakapili Church, one of Honolulu's most prominent and most revered landmarks. At that time the Board members had postponed a decision about burning several buildings between the church and the shacks until they could assess the situation for themselves. But now having completed their own inspections, and feeling ever-increasing pressure to show results, they decided to add those buildings as well to the fire department's list.

Even as the doctors were formally approving these new burn orders, Henry Howard, an eye, ear, nose, and throat physician who ran the city's public dispensary, burst unceremoniously and unexpectedly into the office. The startled Board members turned in surprise to see their friend in evident distress. "The steeple of the Kaumakapili Church has caught fire," Howard blurted out, "and the flames are threatening the whole of Chinatown."[1]

Wood abruptly suspended the meeting, and the three doctors headed immediately in the direction of the church, which was roughly ten blocks away. They found themselves moving through the streets with thousands of other Honolulu residents, drawn by a combination of curiosity and horror, toward a rising billow of sparks, embers, and dense black smoke at the upper end of Chinatown. While guards halted ordinary citizens at the Chinatown quarantine line along Nuuanu Street, Emerson, Day, and Wood rushed on into the plague district. There they found the magnificent twin steeples of Kaumakapili Church roaring with flames like a pair of giant candles and all of the buildings for three adjoining blocks, including those they had just finished condemning back at the office, fully engulfed and blazing uncontrollably. In the midst of the chaos that confronted them, the doctors tried to piece together what had happened.

Fire chief James Hunt had chosen that tranquil Saturday morning as a safe time to burn the condemned shacks in block 15. In the chief's mind, the light offshore breeze and balmy weather conditions minimized any danger of harming nearby Kaumakapili Church, which he certainly did not want to do. Indeed, he had ordered every member of his well-trained and professionally paid fire department to assist in this operation, and he had all four of his fire engines standing by at strategic spots near the church. After thorough consultation with his assistants and careful calculations of wind direction, the chief himself had ignited the shacks at 9:00 A.M.

By all accounts, the fire had begun exactly as planned. The flames moved slowly and predictably in the direction that Hunt had anticipated—away from the church—incinerating the condemned shacks in an orderly manner. After about an hour, however, the morning's light ocean breezes died down, and a far more powerful wind from the opposite direction suddenly began to plunge down off the *pali*. Within minutes, the strong downdrafts, like a giant invisible bellows, abruptly transformed what had been a well-controlled burn into something resembling an open blast furnace, complete with a roaring fountain of embers that rose hundreds of feet into the air. The shift in conditions took place so fast that the firefighters had no chance to extinguish the burning shacks. Instead, they concentrated their hoses on Kaumakapili Church, now downwind from the intensifying fire and directly in harm's way.

The point of no return came when a wind-blown ember ignited Kaumakapili's eastern steeple at a level higher than the fire department's strongest engine could propel water. The flames moved quickly down into the main sanctuary, where they ignited immense piles of clothing that had been collected in the church for fumigation and disinfection as part of the antiplague campaign. While the firefighters concentrated on saving the church, flames spread to nearby structures and were driven by the relentless *pali* winds across the street to the next block. Hundreds of flaming embers floated elsewhere through the upper end of Chinatown, lighting countless spot fires wherever they came to rest. Residents did their best to extinguish these fires, but some were inaccessible and many were far from water supplies. Even as the three physicians arrived, firefighters at the front of the church were forced to abandon their engine to the flames or die themselves. In desperation, they ordered the dynamiting of nearby buildings to create a fire break, but the windblown flames simply jumped over the gap.

For the next several hours, the three Board of Health physicians could do little but watch as the fire front roared through the core of Chinatown's closely packed two-story wooden buildings. Unable to check the flames with the limited equipment they had left, firemen concentrated instead on evacuating people ahead of the advancing conflagration. The intense heat melted iron machinery into molten puddles and baked the earth into ceramic ground covers beneath the flaming structures. A warehouse full of fireworks awaiting the Chinese New Year, just nine days away, exploded in destructive splendor. Stacked lumber near construction sites made spectacular pyres. The loudly hissing wall of flames, still driven by the strong *pali* winds, moved relentlessly down through the quarantined district all the way to the edge of Honolulu's main harbor, where waterborne firefighting equipment managed to keep it from turning east into the commercial center of the city. During the rest of the afternoon, the most densely built and densely populated section of Honolulu burned itself out. By evening the hollow facade of Kaumakapili Church loomed like a medieval ruin over roughly thirty-eight acres of ashen desolation. The area looked as if nothing but the church had ever been there.

In addition to the physical destruction of almost one-fifth of the city's buildings, the great fire also stripped at least five thousand people—more than an eighth of the city's population—of their homes, their businesses, and all the personal possessions they were unable to carry. Roughly half the victims were Chinese; the rest were predominately Japanese and Hawaiian. Few of the refugees felt any loyalty to the government that had placed Emerson, Day, and Wood in charge of the public's health. On the contrary, many of them suspected that the day's fire was a white plot to ruin or even to exterminate them. Everything they had worked so hard to accumulate had been obliterated, and they realized they would now be completely at the mercy of the very authorities who had been ordering the fires in the first place. By the end of the day, many of the district's residents were clearly in shock as the enormity of what happened and the desperation of their own situations began to sink in. Somewhat miraculously, no one had been killed in the disaster. But the day's events had instantly disrupted thousands of lives to an extent no one could have imagined when they awoke that balmy morning.

To make matters worse, everyone inside the Chinatown district had already been under strict quarantine as part of the physicians' campaign to contain the epidemic. As the fire continued to expand, Honolulu citizens from outside the quarantined zone massed on the periphery of Chinatown. They were determined to prevent a general dispersal of the residents trapped inside the district, fearing they might carry the plague uncontrollably throughout the city. Consequently, all of the refugees would now have to be confined in detention camps to make sure they were not carrying the disease. In addition to the consequences of the great fire, after all, Honolulu still had an epidemic of bubonic plague on its hands.

Emerson, Day, and Wood spent the rest of the night trying to respond to the short-term consequences of the catastrophe. Order had to be restored to the city and thousands of terrified people, who were already under armed guard, had to be fed, housed, and resettled. As a smoldering glow illuminated drifting nighttime clouds, the three physicians began to face the fact that a policy they initiated in the name of public health had produced the worst civic disaster in Hawaiian history. The long-term consequences of what had happened could hardly be contemplated.

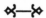

Next to the attack on Pearl Harbor in 1941, the Chinatown fire remains not only the worst civic disaster in Hawaiian history but one of the worst disasters ever initiated in the name of public health by American medical officers anywhere. This book looks at how that catastrophe came about and how the people of Honolulu dealt with it. At its core lies the enduring dilemma of making public health policy in times of crisis on the basis of

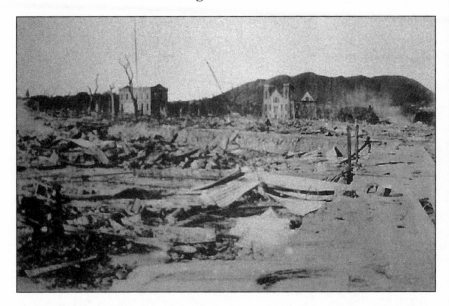

Chinatown after the fire with the ruins of Kaumakapili Church in the distance.
Hawaii State Archives

limited medical knowledge. The three physicians in charge—Emerson, Day, and Wood—rightly remain at the center of this story, and their actions are essential to an understanding of what happened in Chinatown. But this book also demonstrates that their actions and the actions of everyone else involved in this dramatic tale were deeply embedded in a context of racial tensions, cultural assumptions, economic interests, ideological conflicts, medical revolutions, professional rivalries, and American territorial visions. Neither the public health policies developed by the three physicians nor the consequences of those policies can be understood outside their historical context.

1

The World Plague Epidemic
of the 1890s

Few people realize that the world's last major epidemic of bubonic plague occurred quite recently: it began circling the globe at the end of the nineteenth century and killed tens of millions of people worldwide before it receded in the early years of the twentieth century. The disease that Emerson, Day, and Wood were fighting with fire three weeks into the twentieth century had broken out in south-central China sometime before 1870. Severe influenzas and other plague-like diseases were common in that region, but most previous outbreaks had been confined to the interior or had disappeared quite quickly. This new illness, however, seemed to expand and strengthen over time.[1]

By the late 1870s, the disease had decimated most of the provincial villages of south-central China, and by the early 1890s it began appearing along trade routes that led down river valleys toward the coast. Breaking out of the interior, the disease struck the bustling commercial city of Canton with deadly force in 1893, and tens of thousands of people died "like plum blossoms in a late frost." Eyewitnesses remembered that "the dead were buried by the living—and then the living died." Gaining momentum, the epidemic raced rapidly down the heavily traveled Pearl River corridor in 1894 to the port city of Hong Kong, where it began killing the residents of that British coastal colony by the thousands.[2]

The illness typically began with a sudden wave of high fever, headache, chills, and nausea. In many cases, those initial symptoms tapered off after several hours, encouraging victims to hope they had escaped with a mild case of whatever this affliction was. But sometime within the next two days—and often quite quickly—the same symptoms returned more forcefully than before. As their fevers soared to life-threatening levels, victims experienced a crushing combination of overall body pain and almost complete loss of energy. Sufferers often lay limply in a fetal position. Diarrhea, vomiting, lethargy, and mental stupor were common, but not always present, and a bewildering array of other symptoms occasionally appeared as well, including insomnia, speech disorders, delirium, a racing pulse, liver and spleen discomfort, seizures, ruptured blood vessels, and open sores on the skin. Some patients experienced toxic shock and died suddenly after the major onslaught began; others hung on for as many as five unspeakably horrible days, either in semiconscious agony or in a coma, as their internal organs ceased to function and death finally ensued.[3]

The 1894 Hong Kong epidemic had two distinctive traits that seemed to distinguish it from the many previous plague-like diseases and severe influenzas that had regularly appeared there through the nineteenth century. The first was a frighteningly high death rate. Fewer than a quarter of those who came down with the new disease managed to survive. In the British hospitals of Hong Kong, 95 percent of the patients succumbed. Even allowing for the fact that Chinese families took people to those hospitals only as a last resort, that was a devastating death rate for an ailment that now seemed to be spreading so relentlessly and so widely.

The other distinctive symptom of the epidemic was the presence in most victims of badly swollen and exquisitely painful lymph glands, most commonly along the inner thighs and under the armpits. In some patients the swelling at the top of their thighs made their upper legs appear to be inflated. In others the swelling under their armpits gave the impression that a hen's egg was trying to emerge from beneath their shoulder joints. Any pressure on the affected glands—even in cases where the swelling was barely discernible—produced excruciating pain. The few victims who attempted to walk often staggered about in an almost crablike manner to avoid aggravating the pain.

Noting the combination of high death rates and dramatically inflamed glands, which earlier physicians had classically called "buboes," alarmed public health officials in Hong Kong declared the scourge of 1894 to be a return of the legendary bubonic plague, the same affliction that was thought to have killed more than a quarter of the planet's human population during the middle decades of the fourteenth century. From that time through the end of the eighteenth century, recurring waves of the so-called black death—a nickname it acquired because internal hemorrhaging often left dark blotches on its victims' corpses—subsequently killed an estimated fifty million additional people in Europe alone. Though the dreaded disease had apparently never reached the central Pacific or the Western Hemisphere, and for unknown reasons had lapsed into relative quiescence throughout the world near the end of the eighteenth century, it now seemed to be back. Chinese physicians, who knew the black plague as "the great eternal sorrow illness," agreed. Whether this was exactly the same bubonic plague that had ravaged the globe in previous centuries is open to serious debate, but public health officials in the 1890s believed that it was.[4]

The multitude of different symptoms that showed up in different individuals led to widespread medical debates about the fundamental nature of the disease. Was it an intestinal ailment, a skin disease, another of the many fever diseases, or something else altogether? Those debates, in turn, fueled arguments over how best to treat the disease. In the past, plague doctors had tried almost everything, and they were now doing so again. Some attempted to purge their patients' bodies with emetics, hoping to help the body expel whatever was causing the difficulties; some lanced and drained the swollen glands, hoping to relieve the pain and create an exit for internal poisons; some applied salves to inflamed skin as they would for a skin disease; many attempted various methods of fever reduction; and most offered whatever their culture's traditional strengthening and rejuvenating agents might be, which typically included such items as herbal broths, botanical extracts, strong teas, or special foods. But the world's healers all knew full well that they could ultimately do little in the face of bubonic plague except watch and wait helplessly, as their predecessors had done for millennia and the English doctors were still doing in Hong Kong, while the disease ran its horrific and usually fatal course through their patients.

One new development in medical science offered at least some physicians of the 1890s reason to hope—after centuries of frustration—for the possibility of a genuine breakthrough against plague: the rise of bacteriology. During the late 1860s, investigators led by Robert Koch in Berlin and Louis Pasteur in Paris had begun to explore systematically the long-suspected possibility that infectious diseases were caused by extremely tiny creatures that somehow invaded human bodies and disrupted the ability of various organs to function properly. Armed with modern microscopes, investigators were actively searching for such disease-causing microorganisms, all of which were then called bacteria, since the existence of viruses was still unknown. Once identified and isolated, the culprits could be grown in laboratory situations outside the human body, where scientists could work on vaccines, serums, antitoxins, and antidotes to counteract the organisms.

During the 1880s and 1890s, Europeans had used the new bacteriological approach to develop the world's first successful laboratory-produced vaccines and antitoxins, initially and famously against rabies and then even more effectively against diphtheria, which had long been a potent killer of children, and against brucellosis (or undulant fever), a persistent flu-like disease that farmers caught from livestock and city dwellers got from infected milk. Especially for physicians trained in laboratory-oriented medical schools during the last three decades of the nineteenth century, those well-publicized bacteriological triumphs were nothing short of revolutionary. The prospect of more victories to come made scientific medicine in the late 1890s a more optimistic and exciting field than it had ever been before.

Bacteriological investigators around the world were steadily working on many other diseases when the epidemic of 1894 appeared in Hong Kong. Anxious to see if their promising new approach might be applicable to the world's most legendary killer, two prominent investigators rushed to the British colony. One of the two was Kitasato Shibasaburo, who had been sent from his native Japan to work with Koch in Berlin; the other was Alexandre Yersin, who had emigrated from his native Switzerland to France in order to study with Pasteur. Since both of them openly coveted the potential glory of being the first person in history to discover the cause of bubonic plague, the two did not cooperate. Kitasato, for example, tried to prevent Yersin from obtaining bodies to work on. But their rivalry intensified an already frantic research pace. Within months the two scientists more or less simultaneously isolated variations of the same bacterium, which they confirmed to be responsible for the epidemic. Laboratory experiments with animals and pathological reports from the field confirmed the contentions of Kitasato and Yersin that their newly identified pathogen was indeed the perpetrator of bubonic plague.[5]

International public health journals quickly disseminated news of the bacterial discovery that Kitasato and Yersin had made in Hong Kong. The culprit they identified was formally named *pestis*—the plague-producing bacterium—and descriptions of the microorganism circulated the globe, in drawings not unlike wanted posters. Even Honolulu's English-language newspapers published cartoon-like illustrations of what the *pestis* would look like through the lens of a microscope.[6]

Among bacteriologists, the discovery of *pestis* was both exhilarating for its own sake and full of promise for the future. For the first time, physicians knew definitively what was causing bubonic plague, the disease regarded as humankind's most fearsome long-term scourge. By testing for the presence of *pestis* in their patients, physicians could now determine with accuracy whether a suspicious case was that disease. Actual samples of *pestis* were dispatched by ship from Hong Kong to laboratories throughout the world, where medical scientists immediately began trying to produce vaccines, serums, antitoxins, and antidotes to counteract this most recently unmasked bacterial enemy. Physicians and medical students working on the front lines of the global pandemic did the same.

Despite the possibility of long-term progress, however, the discovery of *pestis* in and of itself offered little practical help in the short run for the rank-and-file physicians who actually had to deal with the disease at hand. To make a positive identification, for example, a physician would need a reasonably sophisticated microscope, along with the chemical staining agents that rendered bacteria visible. The physician would also have to know how to obtain and handle human tissue samples, how to prepare those samples properly on a thin pane of glass, and how to discern with confidence exactly what appeared, often dimly and imperfectly, through the eyepiece. In fact, bacteriological equipment and bacteriological skills remained limited around the world through the end of the nineteenth century, so the vast majority of healers continued to diagnose the plague epidemic by its symptoms.

The same was true for treatment. Though bacteriologists in laboratories around the world were already working with their newly acquired samples of *pestis* to develop effective counteragents, no one knew for sure whether their experimental efforts would ever produce useful results, much less how long those efforts might take. In the interim, doctors desperately trying to help actual patients could do nothing more than they were already doing before the discovery.

Nor did the positive identification of *pestis* by itself provide an answer to the question immediately pressing all of the world's public health officers: how and why was this plague continuing to spread? Even if Kitasato and Yersin were right that the disease resulted from the proliferation of *pestis* bacteria inside human bodies, how did the bacteria get there? Did they travel on foul air currents inhaled by unsuspecting victims? Were they ingested with particular foods or bad water? Did they enter human orifices after stowing away on clothing or merchandise? Could they penetrate skin? Might they spread by personal contact?

More than a decade after its appearance in Hong Kong in 1894, scientists would demonstrate that bubonic plague was principally a disease of rodents, especially rats, that was spread from them to humans by the bite of a flea. Whenever a flea sucked blood from a rat that had *pestis* in its bloodstream, the ingested bacteria produced what might be thought of as a throat blockage in the flea. In order to clear its own passageways for fresh blood, the flea essentially vomited the bacterial clot into its next victim, thereby spreading the disease. But no one understood that process in the final years of the nineteenth century.[7]

To be sure, centuries of observation had established a correlation between rat deaths and human deaths in plague epidemics, including this one. Some medical authorities suspected that rats could somehow spread plague once it was underway, perhaps through their fecal matter. That was one of the reasons why British colonial public health officers urged people to wear shoes during the epidemic and one of the reasons why public authorities around the globe had sometimes conducted anti-rat campaigns when plague appeared in past centuries. But most observers either withheld judgment or had concluded that rats, like people, were probably co-victims of plague rather than mobile reservoirs of the disease.

W. J. Simpson, the British public health officer who conducted the British colonial campaigns against plague, maintained through the end of the nineteenth century that rats were no more likely to convey the disease than many kinds of food and many other animals. Walter Wyman, the U.S. federal government's highest-ranking public health officer, published an influential report in 1897 arguing that *pestis* bacteria probably traveled from person to person on dust or foodstuffs; hence rats commonly got the disease because they encountered more dust and more discarded foodstuffs than people did. In a widely circulated magazine that appeared around the English-speaking world in December 1899, a British public health analyst concluded there was "no evidence that rats have been an important factor in spreading infection" during the plague pandemic of the previous five years. After all, reasoned such observers, rats and humans interacted almost everywhere and practically all the time, yet epidemics were infrequent and appeared some places but not others.[8]

Ominously for the rest of the world, the plague that Kitasato and Yersin had studied in Hong Kong soon began to appear in other places as well. With local officials unable to stop it, the disease spread rapidly along trade routes through Southeast Asia. By 1895, people across the Indian subcontinent began dying in record numbers. When major outbreaks of bubonic plague reached the Middle East the following year, nervous European nations began separately to implement quarantines and sanitary measures. Trying to block the epidemic at the border was an ancient and historically ineffective tactic, but it still seemed to be the only defensive strategy available to them. Consequently, the European powers organized an international medical congress in Venice in 1897 to discuss measures that might keep the scourge out of Europe. Since none of the authorities knew exactly what they should be turning away, the protocols allowed for a general scrutiny of goods and people and granted local inspectors a great deal of arbitrary discretion. Even England, a maritime trading nation that had spent the preceding fifty years trying to restrict the use of international quarantines, now ratified the Venetian protocols.[9]

Inside their borders, the European governments launched cleanup campaigns. Public health experts meeting in Berlin to share antiplague strategies reiterated the long-standing categorization of bubonic plague as one of the so-called filth diseases, afflictions that were thought to breed and spread in unclean conditions. Patterns of death throughout China, India, and the Middle East, after all, seemed to reconfirm that opinion, since the dirtiest cities seemed to suffer the highest death rates and people residing in the least sanitary slums of those cities contracted plague in far greater numbers than those living in cleaner neighborhoods.

European public health officials also noticed another characteristic of the epidemic of the 1890s that gave them some hope of avoiding a repetition of what happened when plague devastated their continent in the Middle Ages. Even as hundreds of thousands of Chinese, Southeast Asians, and Indians were dying, European colonial personnel living in the same areas had suffered almost no deaths from the disease. Since even experts did not yet know how plague was transmitted, they did not know that people living in neighborhoods where rats proliferated were more likely to contract the disease than people living in well-manicured areas, such as colonial compounds, or that people wearing long pants and boots, such as colonial officers, were safer from the bites of infected fleas than the urban poor, who generally wore short pants and went about barefoot. Instead, European public health officials drew a conclusion consistent with the pseudoscientific racial theories of that period: they decided that Asians were more susceptible to bubonic plague than Europeans. For that reason, the international protocols ratified at Venice permitted governments to impose separate travel restrictions on some categories of people, such as incoming immigrants from China or India, who seemed more likely to be carriers of the disease, than on other categories of people, such as upper-class whites returning from the same areas.[10]

Many ordinary people in Europe and the United States went even further. To them, the differential death rates indicated that the white race, which they regarded as superior to other races in any event, had happily evolved immunities to what had once been the world's greatest killer. This combination of racial smugness and wishful thinking certainly prevailed among the whites of Honolulu right through the arrival of plague in December 1899. *Austin's Hawaiian Weekly,* for example, assured white Hawaiians that Europeans and Americans living in Asia were so seldom attacked by plague "that no one even discusses the matter." The Honolulu *Independent* reminded residents that plague was not dangerous to whites "who are honest and cleanly." A white housewife writing to friends on the mainland assured them she felt safe because plague "seldom attacks clean white people anyway."[11]

Despite those popular assumptions, public health officers throughout Europe attempted to eliminate the kind of conditions that seemed to enable bubonic plague in Asia, and public health officers throughout the Pacific and the Western Hemisphere expressed concern about their own vulnerability. Since the last major flare-up of bubonic plague more than a hundred years earlier, dramatic changes had taken place in the prevailing patterns of world trade and travel. Many places that had remained relatively isolated through the end of the eighteenth century, and hence relatively safe from all previous epidemics of bubonic plague, were now important nodes on heavily trafficked international routes, and were thus almost certainly more vulnerable in the 1890s than they had been the last time plague spread out of Asia.

Honolulu was just such a place. As late as 1870, most boats coming from the Asian mainland still made the trip to Hawaii under sail power and often took more than two months to get there; by the 1890s, impressive new steam-powered vessels rarely took more than three weeks to make the same trip, even against heavy weather. Hand in hand with improved shipping came increased imperial interest in the Pacific region. England, France, and Germany all wanted a share of the burgeoning Asian trade, and so did the rapidly emerging Japanese empire. Honolulu, which had grown very slowly through the first three quarters of the nineteenth century, found itself strategically in the middle of the increasing trade and naval activity that began vigorously crisscrossing the Pacific in unprecedented volume after 1885. From that point on, the city's population had been rising dramatically.[12]

By 1899 Honolulu was home to just under forty-five thousand people, more than three times its population only twenty years earlier. What had

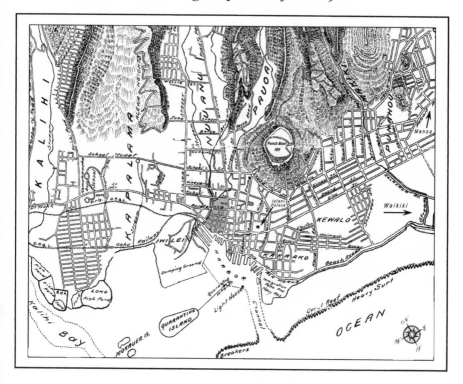

Honolulu at the end of the nineteenth century. Chinatown is shaded. Also note Quarantine Island.

recently been a large town occupying the gently sloping ground north and east of Honolulu harbor already sprawled several miles to the east and west along extensions of Beretania and King Streets, veered up the Manoa Valley, and crept around the extinct crater that locals called Punchbowl Hill, into the lower portions of the Nuuanu Valley. Although the Chamber of Commerce proudly billed the four-story Judd Building, built in 1898 at the corner of Fort and Merchant Streets, and the 1899 six-story Stangenwald Building next door to it as the city's first "sky scrapers," the vast majority of Honolulu's downtown buildings were two-story stone and wooden structures left over from quieter times. The city maintained its unpaved streets with crushed rock. Horses pulled trolley cars and market carts through the central city, and wealthy residents owned horse-drawn carriages, but bicycles were the most common mode of mechanical transportation. Honolulu would not have internal combustion automobiles for sale until 1900.[13]

With ships from all over the world coming and going on a daily basis, the people of Honolulu recognized their city's increased vulnerability to epidemic diseases. Soon after receiving word in 1894 that bubonic plague was spreading outward from Hong Kong, the Honolulu Board of Health had imposed a regimen of inspections and quarantines upon all incoming ships. Shortly thereafter, the Hawaiian government also began maintaining sanitary officers of its own in the principal ports of China and Japan, officers who were charged with inspecting the contents and personnel aboard all vessels outbound for Hawaii. Without a clean bill of health from one of those inspectors, ships from plague ports were summarily denied entry to Honolulu harbor. Even with a clean bill of health, all ships entering Honolulu harbor from ports known to have suffered plague attacks were detained for seven days on a shoal designated as Quarantine Island. Captains had to certify the continuing health of their crews and passengers; violators were subject to a five-thousand-dollar fine and seizure of their ship. Anyone who appeared ill was isolated until the ailment resolved itself.[14]

Though not especially rigorous and ultimately subject to circumvention by unscrupulous captains, that system seemed to be effective. Plague had appeared regularly on other Pacific islands after 1895, but not in the Hawaiian archipelago. In 1896, United States Army medical observers stationed at Pearl Harbor, which had been leased to the American navy, reported back to Washington that nearby Honolulu remained a reasonably salubrious city with a strong and effective Board of Health securely in place and doing a good job. The Honolulu press praised their government's medical defenses, and through the summer of 1899 Hawaii remained plague-free.[15]

2

The "Existing Government" of Hawaii

The government guarding Hawaii from the world pandemic of plague was a watchful and wary one—and not just in matters of public health. Self-proclaimed as the Republic of Hawaii, it was run by a white minority and represented no more than a quarter of the archipelago's population in any meaningful sense. The precarious nature of that government and the still-vivid memory of recent political struggles strongly influenced the behavior and reactions of everyone involved in the great Chinatown fire of January 1900.[1]

Through most of the nineteenth century, the Hawaiian Islands had been ruled by Hawaiian kings. With the permission of those monarchs, Europeans and European Americans gradually but steadily settled in the archipelago, introduced plantation agriculture, and directed international trade. Whites gained additional influence through close counseling relationships with the indigenous aristocracy and successful Christian missionary work. Sugar became the principal source of revenue for the islands, especially after favorable trade treaties were signed with the United States in 1875. In order to increase production of that lucrative crop, the Hawaiian monarchy had permitted whites to import labor—chiefly from China through the 1880s, and then from Japan during the 1890s, but also from such places as the Portuguese Azores. Though legally regarded as foreign citizens, Asians altogether constituted a majority of the archipelago's population by the mid-1890s.

Beginning in the 1880s the sometimes uneven but largely cooperative relationship between the Hawaiian monarchy and the islands' powerful white elites began to break down. Fearful of becoming a colonial figurehead, King David Kalakaua encouraged a renaissance of Hawaiian culture to offset the influence of white outsiders. He also began to exploit rifts in the ranks of the white elites to maintain his own independence. Increasingly led by Americans, the dominant faction of whites formed a rough working alliance of sugar planters, old missionary families, and influential Honolulu merchants to resist what they regarded as the king's irresponsible abuses of power. Accusing Kalakaua of making dangerously arbitrary decisions and awarding government posts to the highest bidders, the white alliance engineered the adoption of a revised constitution in 1887. The new system preserved the monarchy but sharply curtailed the independent prerogatives of the sovereign. The new system also retained many features of the traditional Hawaiian caste system, especially those features that had morphed into white privileges through business arrangements or intermarriage with the Hawaiian aristocracy. And the new constitution of 1887 continued to explicitly exclude virtually all Asians from participation in the political system.

In 1891 Queen Liliuokalani replaced King David Kalakaua on the Hawaiian throne. To the dismay of most whites, she promptly began to reassert traditional sovereignty in ways that directly threatened their privileged economic positions. In the view of many white Americans, Liliuokalani seemed bent upon the counterproductive task of restoring a backward and corrupt form of aristocratic rule. If the queen's counterreformation succeeded, whites feared a period of chaos and destabilization that might make the strategically located Hawaiian islands easy prey for any number of ambitious imperial forces in the Pacific. By 1892, pro-American Honolulu merchants and pro-American sugar planters began meeting in clandestine sessions reminiscent of the Committees of Correspondence that preceded the American Revolution. The name they gave themselves reflected their ultimate goal: the Annexation Club.

The white elites decided by the end of 1892 that the best future for Hawaii, and not incidentally for themselves, could be secured by executing a four-step plan. First, they would have to remove the volcanic Liliuokalani, whom they feared to be dangerously unpredictable. Next they would establish a provisional government to keep the peace and conduct affairs of state in the short term. Third, they would promptly arrange for the voluntary surrender of their provisional government to a speedy annexation by the United States. Finally, they would arrange to have the United States government formally reconstitute the Hawaiian Islands as an American territory. They believed their four-step plan would preserve white control at the local level, while allowing the archipelago to develop under the foreign power of their own choosing—the United States.

The motives of the pro-American annexationists have been debated for more than a century and were probably as varied as their members. Some among them were simply trying to hold on to a cushy situation. Their economic clout had allowed them, in effect, to replace the indigenous aristocracy, and they did not wish to be unseated. Others had persuaded themselves that American-style management of public affairs offered the best chance in the long run for improving the lives of everyone in the islands, not just the whites. The so-called missionary wing of the annexationist movement hoped to see Hawaii become a beacon of Protestant values, beaming brightly at the crossroads of the Pacific. In their view, such an outpost of Christian virtue could best be defended by the United States. According to a later investigation conducted by Democratic congressman James Blount of Georgia, still others in the annexationist camp hoped that an American takeover would restore favorable trading terms for Hawaiian sugar, something that had recently been lost under United States tariff revisions.

Most of the annexationists were also overtly racist and patently paternalistic in their motivations. The white Americans believed they possessed the world's best forms of government, best forms of religion, and best forms of economic development. They regarded Hawaiians, not to mention the islands' Asian majorities, as incapable of enlightened and progressive self-rule, at least under their current circumstances. Consequently, by white logic, the engineering of an American takeover assumed the status of a sacred duty. If the annexationists failed to put Hawaii on the right path while they still could, everyone on the islands was likely to suffer in the future. The guilt for such needless suffering would be upon the eternal consciences of those who saw their duty but failed to act. Though no doubt sincere, white attitudes were breathtakingly arrogant.

In January 1893, Liliuokalani publicly suspended the constitution of 1887 and dramatically announced from the balcony of the Iolani Palace her intention to establish a constitution of her own. Her plan of government would restore indigenous control over the islands and reestablish autocratic royal rule. The Annexation Club, now somewhat augmented in numbers and calling itself the Committee of Safety, took the queen's bold maneuvers as a pretext for launching the four-step plan they had been discussing. The pro-American revolutionaries had previously secured the proactive collusion of the United States minister to Hawaii, a political appointee named John Stevens. Stevens promptly ordered U.S. Marines into the city. Though ostensibly present to protect United States property in what appeared to be an unsettled political situation, the troops were regarded by everyone in Honolulu as a shield for the annexationists.

The palace coup that followed was all but bloodless, since the bulk of the city's white working classes rallied in support of the pro-American elites, while the queen's potential allies dared not confront the marines. Many people in Honolulu seem to have been simply confused and understandably cautious, reluctant to commit themselves forcefully either for or against the contending factions, since neither side could claim untainted legitimacy or anything resembling a general consensus. Though little more than a loosely cooperating network of friends and associates, the pro-American planters and merchants held Liliuokalani under house arrest and declared themselves the provisional rulers of Hawaii.

The Committee of Safety immediately established ruling councils and installed Sanford Ballard Dole as their titular head and provisional president. Most observers, however, considered Lorrin A. Thurston to be the chief architect and guiding spirit of the annexationist takeover. Both men were United States–educated lawyers with strong social and economic ties to the leading white families of Hawaii. As a political team, they complemented each other nicely. Dole's Hawaiian birth, missionary background, Hawaiian-language fluency, Sunday-school-teacher demeanor, and firmly confident sense of high principle made him an ideal and disarmingly resolute front man. Thurston's frequently demonstrated ability to make things happen, combined with his reputation as a brilliant analyst and a man of uncannily shrewd judgment, made him the perfect political strategist. Both men would also be deeply involved seven years later in the events that led to the Chinatown fire.[2]

To follow through with their original intentions, leaders of the provisional government presented themselves the day after the coup to American minister Stevens and asked formally that the islands be placed under the protection of the United States. Playing his prearranged role, Stevens instantly recognized the revolutionaries as the legitimate government of Hawaii, despite the fact that no real government yet existed. Though Stevens lacked legal authority from Washington to take any of these actions, he then ordered the American flag raised over Hawaiian government buildings as a sort of interim acknowledgment of pending annexation.

By the middle of February, the cooperating parties in Honolulu had drafted a treaty designed to make the annexation official.

When news of the Honolulu coup and the proposed treaty of annexation reached Washington, many politicians in the American capital expressed grave misgivings about what seemed to be going on in the Pacific. Democratic congressmen in particular took a dim view of Stevens's behavior. Since the administration he served, that of President Benjamin Harrison, had been defeated in the November elections of 1892, Stevens was a lame-duck Republican appointee at the time he was taking these extraordinary actions. To many Democrats, Stevens's support for the coup and his precipitous and clearly premeditated gestures of recognition looked like flagrant acts of last-minute cronyism on the part of an officer who would be replaced in March, rather than careful steps of statecraft undertaken in the interests of the nation he was supposed to be serving. Consequently, the Democrats successfully delayed action on the proposed Hawaiian treaty and sent Congressman Blount to the islands to determine what was happening six thousand miles from Washington. Democrats thus ensured that their own incoming administration under Grover Cleveland would make the call regarding American relations with Hawaii.

When President Cleveland received Blount's report, he renounced Stevens's actions and apologized for the unauthorized complicity of United States military forces in the coup. To redress the wrong, Cleveland both rejected the proposed annexation and instructed his new minister to Hawaii to lay the groundwork for restoring Liliuokalani to the throne, provided she accepted certain conditions, including amnesty for the revolutionaries. After initially refusing, Liliuokalani apparently acceded to those conditions, but the annexationists in any event adamantly refused to surrender the power they were now consolidating. Since the queen's position on amnesty was disputed, and since American military intervention would look to the rest of the world like de facto annexation anyway, Cleveland decided to do nothing.

With their plan for speedy annexation on hold, Dole and his associates in the provisional government now found themselves in the awkward position of having to put a full-scale and at least semi-permanent domestic government of their own into place if they hoped to remain in power. The revolutionaries did this by drafting yet another new constitution and declaring themselves the Republic of Hawaii. Cleveland felt he had no choice but to recognize the Dole regime, which he did a month later. Liliuokalani, for her part, planned to tour the United States in search of support for restoring her monarchy.

The new Republic of Hawaii was not designed as a long-term solution to the governmental problems of the archipelago; it was designed to maintain the power of a relatively small minority of pro-American leaders until political circumstances in the United States might allow them to secure the final two aims of their original four-step plan: American annexation and territorial status. Consequently, the supporters of the new republic had no intention of risking a fully representative system of government, which they might not be able to control. Even with the support of the American-born working classes, especially in Honolulu, and of the Portuguese, who self-consciously cast their lots with the pro-American oligarchy and thereby successfully "whitened" themselves from marginal foreign laborers to loyal citizens, the new regime could probably count on active political support from less than a quarter of the people then living in the islands.[3]

Under the Dole constitution, Hawaiians could participate in the affairs of the new republic if they renounced the monarchy. A few did so, and they cast their lots with the annexationists. According to the Hawaiian opposition, indigenous supporters of the new regime believed that the promise of prosperity and protection under the wing of the United States outweighed the perils of trying to retain an already doomed independence. Many other Hawaiians continued in their government jobs, which included police work, and continued to serve under the new republic in the Hawaii National Guard, even while remaining passively loyal to the old monarchy and uninvolved in the actual politics of the Dole administration. Still others remained deeply and openly resentful of what they continued to characterize as "the arrogant Republic of Hawaii, which hands the nation over for America to snatch."[4]

Though Chinese and Japanese residents together comprised more than half of Hawaii's total population by the time of the coup, they had already been denied citizenship under the constitution of 1887. The new Dole administration had no desire to involve Asians in its annexationist government either. In fact, the Dole administration could hardly have gotten off to a worse start in the eyes of Hawaii's Asians.

Within a month of seizing power, the postrevolutionary provisional government began publicly discussing two proposals that the Chinese population in particular found outrageous. One was a bill that would have prevented anyone brought into the islands as an agricultural laborer from ever changing occupations. An earlier version of that proposal had been debated and rebuffed by the Hawaiian government in 1889, but its largely American backers sensed a fresh opportunity under the new annexationist regime. The other would have required any Asian person who wanted to engage in trade or manufacture to acquire a license not required of whites. Moreover, such licenses would be available only to those Chinese who were already engaged in trade or manufacture; no new licensees would be permitted.[5]

Together, the proposals illuminated both the anti-Asian biases and the flagrant self-interests of the merchant-planter alliance that supported the coup. The same planters who wanted Hawaii to become a United States territory—the sooner the better—realized that they would no longer be free to import laborers from the Asian mainland once their goal was actually achieved; as an American possession, Hawaii would fall under the United States's infamous Chinese Exclusion Acts, which would effectively bar future immigration. Consequently, the planters were exploring ways to prevent Chinese workers who were already there from leaving the fields for jobs in towns and cities, as they had been doing in large numbers after their field contracts expired. Once in towns and cities, moreover, especially in Honolulu itself, the Chinese were vigorously building strong networks of diversified businesses and competing successfully with their English-speaking rivals in a host of trades as diverse as construction and accounting. By the 1880s, enterprising Chinese businessmen controlled more than a quarter of Honolulu's wholesale commerce and more than half its retail activity. As a result, some of the pro-American merchants had joined the planters in support of the Asians-in-agriculture policy, and then added the license idea as a way to handicap the competition.[6]

Discussion of these proposals was met with instant outrage in the increasingly active and well-organized Chinese business community of Honolulu. Chinese leaders in the city quickly mustered a mass meeting of more than two thousand Chinese who vehemently and publicly protested further action on any such policies. Presiding at the meeting was Lau Chung, who controlled the powerful Wing Wo Tai Company. Aligned with Lau were the men who managed Honolulu's largest Chinese businesses: Ah Leong, a merchant and investment broker; Wong Chow, whose Yee Wo Chan Company was a leading importer of Asian goods; and the partners Hong Quon and Sing Chang, who controlled the financially strong Sing Chong investment company. These international businessmen had much to lose if the new government succeeded in crippling their activities.[7]

"By what right do our white-skinned brothers assume to lord it over us, and to say that we shall do business, and trade, and live and breathe, only by their consent?" demanded one of the speakers at the mass rally. Another hinted that such actions on the part of the whites might force the

Chinese to find "a man of war" among themselves in the future. The audience called for unity and action. At the end of the rally, a delegation was chosen to convey a unanimous resolution of protest to the provisional government. In the volatile atmosphere of the immediate postcoup period, the Dole administration decided that discretion was the better part of valor and quietly backed off. But the fact that the new government had seriously entertained the two proposals at all planted poisonous seeds of enduring suspicion in the Chinese community from the very first months of Dole's provisional rule.[8]

Japanese residents in Hawaii, whose numbers were rising dramatically, took the occasion of the annexationist coup to demand access to citizenship in the new republic. This put the founders of the Dole republic on the horns of dilemma, especially since that demand had the strong and official support of Japan's rapidly modernizing and muscle-flexing home government. On the one hand, the annexationists did not want to share citizenship with any of Hawaii's Asians, including the Japanese, or worse, risk an Asian takeover of the islands by majority vote. On the other hand, because the annexationists initially planned to continue to import Japanese labor, they did not want to alienate the Japanese home government either. The annexationists solved their problem by dropping the explicit ban on Asian citizenship from the previous Hawaiian constitution and inserting an English-and-Hawaiian literacy test for citizenship into the new republican constitution. This solution allowed Japanese officials to claim they had forced the removal of discriminations based specifically on ethnicity, even though everyone realized that almost all Asians, including the Japanese, would continue to be excluded from the political process by almost absurdly rigid enforcement of the new literacy clause.

Rather than risk a referendum on the proposed constitution, the pro-American oligarchy proclaimed its new republic at a mass rally of ratification, a rally well guarded by loyal troops. In an obvious nod toward the United States, Dole and his allies inaugurated their government on July 4, 1894, and proceeded to fill its various committees and offices with trusted friends and allies from the Annexation Club and the Committee of Safety. Among the new republic's officially constituted public agencies was a Board of Health, staffed with a mix of Western-trained physicians and prominent civilians, who reported to the attorney general. That agency was charged with protecting Hawaii from the world pandemic of bubonic plague.

After six months of uneasy rule, the Dole government in Honolulu faced an open attempt at counterrevolution in January 1895. The insurrection was loosely organized and haphazardly led by a small cadre of dissidents. Many of the insurgents had lost positions of influence or economic advantage when the monarchy had fallen. All of them resented the annexationists allied with Dole, who seemed bent upon delivering their homeland to the United States. The rebels were joined by a motley collection of other Dole opponents, including some Hawaiians loyal to Liliuokalani and a few disappointed office seekers from the republican camp. The purported royalists, who had earlier secreted weapons and whispered conspiratorial words of uprising, invaded Honolulu from Diamond Head. They hoped their armed resistance would serve as a leaven to foment popular unrest. Instead, the tiny and ineffective force was quickly driven into the hills above the city and eventually rounded up by much-stronger militia units organized by the Dole government. In the aftermath, Liliuokalani was compelled to sign a formal document of abdication.

Suppression of the embarrassingly inept effort at open rebellion made Dole's republic appear both stronger and more legitimate than it probably was, but did little to dampen distrust between the government and Honolulu's Asians. Some Chinese had helped provide supplies for the government's volunteers, but most were suspected of sympathizing with, and perhaps even directly aiding, the counterrevolutionaries. One of the chief rebel leaders, the half-Hawaiian royalist Robert William Kalanihiapo Wilcox, had close ties by marriage to leading Hawaiian Chinese families. Oral traditions in Honolulu's Chinese community for the next fifty years sustained the belief that Chinese merchants had indeed helped underwrite the counterrevolution, annoyed as they were with the alliance between their American competitors and the Dole regime. Decades after the affair, some elderly Chinese even claimed to remember seeing the bodies of two suspected rebels lying in the streets of Chinatown, victims of a shoot-out with Dole militia. Whether those memories were literally accurate, they attested to the enduring antipathy of many Honolulu Chinese toward Dole's Republic of Hawaii.[9]

In March 1897, the Republican William McKinley was inaugurated as president of the United States. The change in the Washington administration encouraged Dole and the other leading annexationists to resume their original efforts to secure a formal takeover of Hawaii by the United States. The Hawaiian Republic's representatives in Washington developed close relations with key officials in the new administration, particularly naval officials; the Hawaiian legislature sent Dole himself to Washington to plead the annexationists' case. The indefatigably effective Lorrin Thurston articulated the case for American takeover in an influential publication entitled *A Hand-book on the Annexation of Hawaii*, which—among other things—convincingly rebutted Congressman Blount's earlier dismissal of the annexationists' coup as little more than a sugar planters' plot.[10]

Even with the support of the administration, however, those in favor of annexation could not command a two-thirds vote in the United States Senate. This was a serious impediment because annexation had been presented in the form of a treaty between the Republic of Hawaii, which had been recognized by the Cleveland administration, and the United States; and treaties required a two-thirds vote of the Senate for ratification. To circumvent that constitutional problem, annexationist forces maneuvered to have Hawaii taken over by joint resolution of both houses of Congress, as Texas had been in the 1840s. That would require the representatives as well as the senators to approve the takeover, but it could be achieved with simple majorities in the two chambers.

A majority in the House of Representatives approved the joint resolution on June 15, 1898, and a majority in the Senate followed suit three weeks later. Both votes were strongly influenced by the U.S. declaration of war on Spain just two months earlier. Since military conflict was already underway in the Philippines, secure possession of the Hawaiian archipelago seemed strategically prudent. When news of the joint resolution reached Honolulu, the Dole government publicly rejoiced at the curiously paradoxical triumph of having given away the independent autonomy of everyone in Hawaii, including themselves. From then on, Hawaii would be a possession of the United States. Only the fourth step of the annexationists' plan remained to be taken: the installation of a formal territorial government.

To the dismay of Dole and his associates, Congress did not immediately take that final step. Many Americans had grave doubts about affording the Hawaiian Islands—with their overwhelmingly nonwhite population and their two-thousand-mile distance from the rest of the nation—the same constitutional status that Americans had granted to contiguous North American territories acquired earlier in the century, a status that strongly implied the possibility of future statehood. Recognizing the strength of such doubts, hesitant politicians in Washington initially blocked all proposals to install a standard territorial regime. Instead, Congress settled into a prolonged debate over the legal status of the nation's newest possession, a debate that would continue into the summer of 1900.[11]

Anticipating such a contingency, the joint resolution of annexation had stipulated that "the existing government" in Hawaii would continue to exercise "civil, judicial, and military powers," subject to the authority and direction of the president of the United States, "until Congress shall provide for the government of such islands." Moreover, "the municipal legislation of the Hawaiian Islands" would also "remain in force until the Congress of the United States shall otherwise determine."[12] In other words, the Dole administration would remain in place and continue to function under its own local laws until the territorial debate was resolved in Washington. Though President McKinley was ultimately responsible for the archipelago, even the United States naval forces at Pearl Harbor continued to deal with the preexisting Dole administration as if it was still an independent authority. As a result, when the world pandemic of bubonic plague finally appeared in Honolulu in the final months of 1899, the white minority Dole administration was going to have to deal with it, whether they wanted to or not.

3

The Arrival of *Pestis*

W hen the *Nippon Maru* dropped anchor in Honolulu harbor in June 1899, its captain told the Board-appointed physician who rowed out to inspect the ship that he had a dead body below decks. A Chinese passenger had died at sea a few days before, said the captain, and since he was scheduled to go next to San Francisco, he wanted to off-load the body in Honolulu so the victim's remains could be returned to China. Though the ship's own doctor had already certified the cause of death as uremia, a toxic blood poisoning, the Hawaiian government health inspector had his doubts. So before granting permission for anything or anyone to come ashore, the inspector asked his superiors on the Board of Health what to do.

Francis Day, one of the Board's three physicians, came down to the harbor to see for himself. Day boarded the vessel, carefully inspected the body, and took some tissue samples from the dead passenger. When he got back to his office, he gave some of the tissue samples to Dr. Luis Alvarez, a friend in private practice who had recently taken a course on basic bacteriological methods. Day then discussed his notes and observations with his medical colleagues on the Board of Health. On the basis of the telltale signs that Day reported, they all concluded that the Chinese passenger had almost certainly died of plague, not uremia. Consequently, Day clamped severe restrictions on the *Nippon Maru*. The ship would wait at Quarantine Island for seven days. No one could disembark and no cargo could be landed.[1]

Alvarez reported the next day that he was pretty certain he could see plague bacilli in the tissue samples Day had given him. But he could not be sure: this was his first solo effort at bacteriological sleuthing. Fortunately for everyone aboard the *Nippon Maru*, no additional cases appeared during the week they spent tethered to Quarantine Island. As a result, Day and his colleagues saw no reason to alarm the public. Instead, the doctors on the Board of Health quietly decided to let the ship depart for San Francisco, provided the captain agreed to carry a cautionary warning to that city's health inspectors. Only a few people in Honolulu were even aware of the passenger's death, and the city's newspapers continued to express confidence in the ability of Hawaii's medical defenses to hold the worldwide plague epidemic completely at bay.[2]

Although Hawaii's health inspectors paid close attention to people and goods, as evidenced in the *Nippon Maru* incident, they paid no particular attention to the possibility of rats escaping from incoming ships. Since those rodents and their fleas were not yet recognized as the principal purveyors of the plague, no one thought to worry about them. The Honolulu Board of Health would later require crews to put rat-blocking devices on the ropes they used to tie their vessels to the city's wharves. That requirement, however, was imposed only after plague was already rampant inside the city; and ironically, the precaution was ordered "not for our protection [ashore]," Board of Health president Wood later explained, "but for theirs," to protect the crews on ships from potentially plague-carrying rats in Honolulu.[3]

Whether from the *Nippon Maru* or from another ship—some Chinese later suspected that plague had come in with foodstuffs aboard the steamship *Manchuria*—at least one plague-infected rat almost certainly entered Honolulu sometime between June and August of 1899. Through October and into November, the disease spread steadily among the city's rats, particularly those living close to the wharves, as infected rat fleas jumped from rodent to rodent. The residents of lower Chinatown noticed unusually large numbers of dead rats in the area just above the harbor. Rat fleas prefer to travel among rats, and normally jump to humans only occasionally. But as more and more rats succumbed, desperate rat fleas began to turn to any available warm-blooded hosts, including humans.[4]

By late fall, rumors of a deadly new disease began to circulate inside the Chinese community. All of those struck down had lived in the lower part of Chinatown, adjacent to the harbor. Traditional Chinese healers were divided over what the new disease might be and how they should deal with it. They knew that bubonic plague had been stalking the globe for five years, and they recognized the ominous character of the cases breaking out around them, especially the fact that most of those suffering had badly swollen glands. But the traditional healers generally preferred to categorize the mysterious new malady either as some variation of the so-called seasonal sicknesses (*shi zheng*) they had long associated with old China or as the return of what elderly Chinese called the "giddy illness." To treat the new affliction, herbalists boiled indigo root (*banlan gen*, or Chinese woad), which patients drank as an antitoxin and applied as a warm compress on their swollen glands. As news of the disease spread throughout Chinatown, however, many nervous residents of the district quietly began to relocate, moving their possessions with them to other areas of the city.[5]

The residents of Chinatown had good reason to deal quietly with the new disease among them. Four years earlier, shortly after the current government had overthrown the Hawaiian monarchy and established itself as the Republic of Hawaii, a rash of sudden deaths had occurred on the edge of Chinatown. American physicians then serving on the new government's Board of Health tentatively diagnosed the fatal cases as cholera, but most Chinese healers and a few Westerners disagreed. Since identification of the distinctive comma-shaped cholera bacillus had been one of Koch's triumphs in the 1880s, the Americans had a way to settle the dispute. But no one in Honolulu in 1895 knew enough about bacteriological analyses to conduct the necessary examinations locally, so they had to dispatch bacterial samples to laboratories in the United States for verification.

Rather than wait several weeks for the results, the new government decided to act on the assumption that their own physicians' diagnosis was correct. Evoking emergency powers, the Board of Health sealed off the affected districts in an effort to contain the outbreak. Business was suspended within the sealed districts; schools were closed; and all public meetings, even church services, were banned. Board members also enlisted other physicians and civilian volunteers to inspect each person in the quarantined districts twice a day. Though the United Chinese Society provided traditional healers from their own community to help perform those inspections, Chinese residents deeply resented the arbitrary invasion of their personal privacy by people they did not know and in many cases with whom they could not even communicate. To make matters worse, any residents who seemed to be coming down with anything were forcibly removed from their homes and taken to a special hospital for

observation and treatment by government-appointed physicians, who practiced a form of medicine most Chinese considered alien and dangerous.[6]

In all of these actions, the American doctors had the complete support
of the newly installed annexationist government. Recently inaugurated
president Sanford Dole candidly observed in a letter to a friend at the end
of July 1895, "cholera has been engrossing our attention for [the] past few
weeks. The Board of Health is the government now . . . and hundreds of
volunteers," he proudly reported, "are carrying out a rigid work of inspecting every house in Honolulu twice a day."[7]

Inside the quarantined districts, the government also implemented a
vigorous cleanup campaign, since the Board's physicians believed that
cholera could spread through contaminated food, bad water, and the ema-
nations associated with rotting organic materials. Though most of the
deaths were occurring among Hawaiians in the Iwilei district, most of the
cleanup efforts took place in the thirty blocks that comprised Chinatown,
which everyone agreed had dreadful sanitary conditions and which, according to the medical assumptions of the day, would be an area of potential disaster if cholera should begin to spread.

Working with the Board of Health and with citizen volunteers, the
residents of Chinatown had hauled tons of human waste, animal remains,
and general garbage out to sea. They scoured privies and applied disinfectants. The Board of Health drafted new requirements for food handling
and for the storage of perishable goods in marketplaces. Relief committees provided meals for penniless workers unable to get out to their jobs,
and the United Chinese Society issued promissory certificates, redeem-
able for medicinals at Chinese drugstores and herbal shops, to residents of
Chinatown unable to afford suggested remedies.

Eighty-five people died before the cholera outbreak abruptly ended.
But the Board's prompt and decisive actions, especially after laboratory
results in the United States confirmed the presence of cholera, were hailed
around the world as a public health triumph, a bold stroke that probably
saved the city from far more devastating losses of life. The sealing-off of
Chinatown and the subsequent cleanup campaign in that district seemed
particularly successful. Yet various groups within Honolulu itself had come
away from the cholera crisis with remarkably different impressions of what
had taken place and hence what they should learn from the experience.[8]

Shortly after it ended, President Dole summarized the 1895 cholera
crisis in positive terms: "The experience which the cholera brought was a
beneficial one in more ways than one," he concluded. "[I]t brought out
conspicuously the fine public spirit that is the chief strength of the Re-

public; it also swamped in some measure the political divisions of the community, and brought many royalists into relations with the government and its supporters in a way which has done them a great deal of good and which may be said to have given them a new horizon." As he so often did, Dole saw "divine sympathy and powerful aid" at work in the health crisis. Successful suppression of a potential cholera epidemic demonstrated to him that he and his recently inaugurated regime were indeed "working to accomplish God's purpose in this country." As long as they sustained what Dole called "a reasonable degree of correctness in [their] conclusions," the new pro-American rulers of Hawaii self-confidently and self-righteously believed they would continue to enjoy the support of the Lord.[9]

In sharp contrast to Dole's impression of widespread cooperation and good will, many Chinese in Honolulu had emerged from the cholera episode convinced that white physicians could not be trusted. Though the Board of Health strongly denied any discrimination, several Chinese patients complained repeatedly about the anti-Asian attitude of Western physicians at Honolulu's temporary cholera hospital. Leaders in the Chinese community believed their countrymen's complaints and concluded that they would have to establish their own hospital to insure better care for their community in the future. Chinatown's largest sociopolitical organizations, the United Chinese Society and the China Engine Company, endorsed a formal petition to the legislature requesting a grant of land for that purpose. No doubt influenced by the fact that the hospital committee was headed by Gu Kim Fui, the legislature ceded the petitioners a parcel in the Palama district just west of Chinatown. In addition to serving as president of the United Chinese Society, Gu Kim Fui was one of the most powerful business leaders in Honolulu. Partly as a consequence of being the city's most prominent Chinese Christian, he also had personal ties to many officials in the Dole administration. Both Chinese and whites contributed to the hospital fund, and by March 1897 the new Chinese hospital at Palama, known as Wai Wah Yee Yuen, opened for patients.[10]

In addition to medical discrimination, the residents of Chinatown also remembered that the policies credited with defeating cholera had left their community financially crippled. A whole season of business had been lost while the district was sealed off from the rest of the city. Overall community income fell drastically when workers could not get out to their jobs. During the cholera crisis, the residents of Chinatown had seen how easily civilian government could be suspended in the face of a medical emergency, how invasive the Board of Health could be when acting unchecked, how quickly people under quarantine could become completely dependent upon the larger community for basic needs, and how shoddily Asians could be treated by white medical volunteers. Consequently, in the opinion of most Chinatown residents and most traditional Chinese healers during the final months of 1899, maintaining extreme discretion with regard to the new disease among them—and even surreptitiously burying the dead—seemed preferable to raising alarms. They did not want a possibly unfounded threat of plague in 1899 to trigger another round of intervention in their lives similar to what they had experienced in 1895.

Also living and practicing inside Chinatown, however, were Chinese physicians who took a strikingly different approach from that of the traditional healers and most of the other residents. At the head of the dissenting faction were Dr. Li Khai Fai and Dr. [Li] Kong Tai Heong, who were married but maintained separate practices. Li Khai Fai had been born into a prominent and scholarly family in a region of south China wracked by political, social, and economic disruption. Most people in the region blamed outside Europeans for their misery, and Li's father had led mobs that stoned European missionaries to death. When Lutherans from Germany subsequently converted the elder Li to Christianity, however, he became a target of the same mobs. At the age of nine, Li Khai Fai had watched in horror as his father, now "a running dog of the white devils," was stoned to death in the street. Li's mother fled with her four children to the relative safety of nearby Hong Kong.[11]

Like her martyred husband, Li's mother believed that Western medicine went hand in hand with Western Christianity as a progressive reform badly needed in China. Consequently, in order to carry forward his legacy, Li's mother enrolled in the Canton Medical School—besides, as she forthrightly acknowledged, she was a widow with four children to feed. Though directed by an American doctor from Ohio, the school had long-standing ties with the Berlin Missionary Society under whose auspices the elder Li had become a Lutheran. As soon as he was old enough, Li Khai Fai followed his mother to the Canton Medical School. He too was determined to sustain his father's legacy of Western-style reform, but he expanded his vision of progress beyond religion and medicine to embrace Western-style political structures as well. At the age of sixteen, he became the radical student leader of a political organization called the Make China Strong Society, which advocated an end to the arbitrary authority of the corrupt and dysfunctional Qing dynasty. Li then left that organization to join a political reform group organized by one of his fellow medical students, Sun Tai Cheong, who had recently returned from Hawaii and who would later be known to the world as Dr. Sun Yat-Sen.[12]

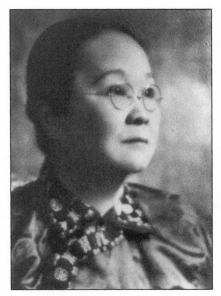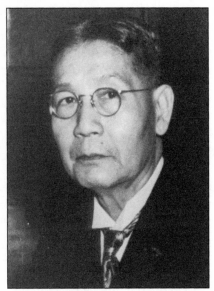

Dr. Kong Tai Heong, left, and Dr. Li Khai Fai. Mamiya Medical Heritage Center. Hawaii Medical Library

While studying at Canton Medical School, the tall and fiery Li met and fell in love with his classmate Kong Tai Heong. Her diminutive size belied the resilience of this forceful and independent-minded young woman, whose route to medical school had been every bit as dramatic as Li's own. Kong had been abandoned as an infant on the doorstep of a Lutheran mission in Hong Kong, with nothing more than her name pinned to the basket in which she was found. Smart and able, she grew up helping the German nuns care for other girls in the orphanage where she lived. The sisters, in turn, arranged for Kong to apply to Canton Medical School, where several of their co-religionists had studied Western medicine. Favorably impressed with this former "basket baby," the faculty admitted her. She immediately excelled and was soon regarded by her professors as the most brilliant medical student in her class.

As students, Li and Kong worked together to master Western medicine with the full commitment of true converts, eagerly embracing the new bacteriological understanding of disease. The most intense period of their training occurred when the plague struck Canton and Hong Kong in 1893 and 1894. Li and Kong often worked around the clock beside their professors, trying to save victims brought into the school's clinic.

Despite their best efforts, most of their patients died horrible deaths before their eyes—and their professors assigned them the grim task of disposing of the dead.[13]

As their graduation approached in June 1896, the two hoped to marry. But their union was initially opposed both by Li's relatives, who did not want his mother's oldest son to marry a woman without a family, and by Kong's professors, who did not want their protégée to run off with a political hothead. The two overcame the objections—Li by arranging to lose the bride his family had selected for him in a card game, and Kong by defying the faculty. But the objections had strengthened the couple's desire to escape to someplace where young professionals could be out from under what they considered the stifling oppression of late-nineteenth-century China, yet still be able to make a difference in the future of Chinese people. They hoped to find such a place in Hawaii, where their friend Sun had gone to school, even though the new government there had recently forbidden incoming Chinese to remain in the islands more than one year.

Li and Kong graduated from Canton Medical School on the morning of June 3, 1896, and were married in a Lutheran chapel that same afternoon. The following day they boarded the *Garrick*, a steamer carrying Chinese merchandise and Asian foodstuffs to Hawaii. Delayed more than a week by unusually heavy storms at sea, the *Garrick* arrived exactly one month later. As they entered Honolulu harbor, Li and Kong heard the sound of artillery fire coming from the center of the city, saw palls of smoke drifting toward them, and wondered fearfully what was going on. Downtown beside the Iolani Palace, the pro-American government was firing ceremonial salutes that day, July 4, to recognize the second anniversary of the Republic of Hawaii.

Li worked the rest of the summer as a common laborer, and the two young physicians lived in abject poverty. With the legal status of temporary aliens, Li and Kong could not practice medicine. At one point, these two would-be reshapers of Chinese culture had to pawn their wedding clothes to buy food. Through a mutual acquaintance, Li and Kong met the Reverend Frank Damon, who had served many years as a missionary in Canton. Kong boldly explained both her plight and her hopes to Damon, who arranged a formal audience for Li with President Dole himself. Li so impressed Dole that the president permitted the two young medical graduates to become permanent residents of the new republic and to open practices. By the end of October, they had obtained formal licenses and set up offices in Chinatown, where they began to build practices that served both Chinese and Hawaiian patients.[14]

The Arrival of Pestis

Between 1896 and 1899, Li and Kong clashed often with Honolulu's traditional Chinese healers. Li in particular made no effort to hide his contempt for the traditional healers, whom he criticized as the unthinking defenders of a backward way of life. The traditionalists, in turn, portrayed their new rivals as traitorous agents of the hostile white devils, dangerous upstarts bent upon displacing centuries of Chinese medical knowledge. That accusation had some merit because Li, Kong, and a few others like them in the Chinese community had more in common professionally with the American physicians on the Honolulu Board of Health than they did with the city's traditional Chinese healers.

Li Khai Fai, in fact, thought that the Chinese in Hawaii should be trying to cooperate not just medically but in all ways with representatives of the United States. Notwithstanding that nation's record of anti-Asian behavior, he believed, American constitutional principles would ultimately protect the Chinese of Hawaii and put them in a position to help their countrymen back home move away from absolutism and superstition toward democratic liberation and scientific reason. For him, cooperation with the American physicians on the Board of Health would be a step forward rather than a concession to oppressors. And possibly because they had not been in Honolulu during the cholera scare, the two Chinese medical graduates had no preexisting skepticism toward their American medical colleagues.[15]

Consequently, when the mysterious plague-like deaths began occurring in Chinatown during the final months of 1899, Li urged residents to report any suspicious cases to the Board of Health rather than explain them away or hide them from public view. In his opinion, bacteriological investigation was the only way to know for sure whether or not the new disease was plague; and if it was, the community had an obligation to mobilize against it. Li and Kong, after all, had already witnessed what this epidemic could do to a city once it gained a secure foothold. They fervently hoped the Chinese residents of Honolulu would do all they could to prevent the plague from devastating their new home as terribly as it had devastated Canton and Hong Kong during their student days.

A series of events beginning on the night of December 11 abruptly ended the internal debates within Chinatown. That evening a manager at the Wing Wo Tai Company, Lau Chung's impressive manufacturing and retail operation in Nuuanu Street, sent one of his employees to find Dr. George Herbert, an English physician who had established a close rapport with the Hawaiians of Maui before coming over to Honolulu as director of the Oahu Insane Asylum. The manager wanted Herbert to examine one of his bookkeepers, twenty-two-year-old You Chong, whose grave symptoms looked to the unhappy merchant suspiciously like the symptoms of the dreaded black death that was rumored to be circulating through the district. Traditional Chinese medications had failed to retard You Chong's decline, and by the time Herbert arrived, the bookkeeper had slipped into a coma. You Chong died at 5:00 A.M. on December 12, 1899. Herbert was convinced, as You's employer had feared, that the patient died of plague.[16]

Before conducting a postmortem, Herbert sent for Dr. Walter Hoffman, a twenty-seven-year-old German physician who had become the city's first official bacteriologist just four months earlier. When word of the autopsy underway at Wing Wo Tai's store spread among Honolulu's physicians, Dr. Duncan Carmichael also joined Herbert and Hoffman. Carmichael represented the United States Marine Hospital Service in Hawaii. If the rumors of plague were true, he would have to report the outbreak to Washington as quickly as possible. Sun Chin, the doctor who had cared for the dead bookkeeper before Herbert's arrival, also witnessed the post mortem, as did Day, who came over to officially represent the Board of Health.

Under the light of kerosene lanterns, the five doctors opened You's corpse and examined his internal organs. Everything they found was consistent with what they knew about bubonic plague. Hoffman prepared slides from the dead man's lymph glands in order to look for the tell-tale *pestis* bacteria, but even before he could put them under his microscope, all the physicians present that morning were reasonably certain on the basis of what they observed during the autopsy that You Chong had died of plague.

From Li Khai Fai, the American physicians departing the Wing Wo Tai building learned that another Chinese bookkeeper had died overnight. Employed at the store of Tam Ping Sam Kee just around the corner in Maunakea Street, forty-year-old Yuk Hoy had been under the care of Tong San Kai, another Western-trained Chinese physician, who now joined Hoffman and the other American doctors at a second impromptu autopsy. They quickly saw that Yuk Hoy too had suffered from badly swollen glands and internal hemorrhaging, the classic symptoms of bubonic plague. Hoffman took tissue samples from Yuk Hoy's remains for bacteriological confirmation, but Yuk's case removed any lingering doubts in the minds of the physicians present: the world epidemic had arrived in Honolulu. And the plague was already spreading. By the end of the day, it would strike down two more Chinese workers and a twenty-seven-year-old man from the Gilbert Islands, all of whom lived in the same neighborhood as the dead bookkeepers.[17]

At noon, the Board of Health convened in emergency session to hear testimony from any doctors who had attended recent fatalities, including Li Khai Fai and other Chinese physicians familiar with Western medicine. With the help of his wife and a Chinese-English medical dictionary, Li prepared a formal report on one of the cases the American doctors had not yet seen. Li's report was a classic description of plague: he found the victim with a high fever, "tossing and trembling like the sea in a typhoon, quaking and quivering, bending and unbending in delirium, like the branches of a tree in thunder and lightning gone crazy." Like the hundreds of plague victims Li and Kong had seen in Canton, the dead man had "the same black spots, . . . the same bleeding through the mouth, the same swellings in the armpits, the groin, . . . the same coma at the end— and then only death." Wood quizzed Li at length about the Honolulu cases, and all three physicians on the Board pressed him for details about the epidemic he had seen firsthand in China. Most of the other physicians summoned for opinions—both Chinese and white—confirmed Li's opinion that Honolulu had bubonic plague on its hands.[18]

Though a few of the doctors present at the emergency session thought that Emerson, Day, and Wood should wait for the report of their own bacteriologist, they themselves had already seen and heard enough. By unanimous vote, the three Board physicians formally declared their city under attack from bubonic plague. They then quickly and unanimously agreed upon a series of policies designed to address the mortal threat now confronting the people of Honolulu. The entire meeting lasted just forty-five minutes.[19]

Under the republic's constitution, the Board's declaration would have created a state of emergency and permitted them to do whatever they deemed necessary during the emergency to protect the public health. But that constitution had been legally suspended in order to facilitate the joint resolution of annexation, so the Board's members were uncertain about the limits of their authority under the "existing government" rules promulgated by the United States Congress. Consequently, they reassembled at three o'clock to confer with the Council of State, which had been Hawaii's highest governmental body under the Dole republic.

The Board's members asked the council to formally confirm their emergency powers and to ratify the policies they had hastily outlined just two hours earlier. Within minutes, the full council not only unanimously confirmed the Board's emergency medical powers but also unanimously ceded absolute control over the entire Hawaiian archipelago to the Honolulu Board of Health for the duration of the plague crisis. Fully convinced that the outbreak of bubonic plague necessitated extraordinary measures, and clearly relieved that an appropriate arm of government had come forward to deal with the situation despite the confusing constitutional circumstances they faced, President Dole and Attorney General Henry E. Cooper agreed that nothing should be allowed to impede the Board of Health's battle against "the dread disease." In a single brief meeting, the civilian government of Hawaii essentially suspended itself.[20]

Thus three physicians found themselves holding absolute dictatorial authority over all aspects of everyday life in Hawaii. They were in command of the armed forces and had unrestricted access to the treasury. They could arbitrarily impose any rules on any subject whatsoever. As one local editor correctly observed, "In this crisis the Board of Health has a greater power than even Congress." And the physicians were clearly expected to exercise their power, since everyone was depending upon them to save the islands, stranded as they were in the middle of the Pacific Ocean, from the nightmare of decimation by plague. Consequently, the newly empowered rulers of Hawaii went immediately from their meeting with the council back across the street to the Board of Health office, where they had recently installed telephones. There they began to implement the policies they had hastily agreed upon just a few hours earlier, policies that would profoundly affect the city for the next several months and beyond.[21]

4

The Government's Plague Fighters

The events of December 12, 1899, abruptly catapulted three physicians to unprecedented positions of absolute power in the Hawaiian Islands. All three had earned their MDs at American medical schools, all three had practiced in the islands for over a decade, and all three had considerable experience as public health officers in Hawaii. But none of them could have imagined becoming rulers of the archipelago—not just in matters of health but in economic, social, and all other matters as well. In a literal sense, and almost literally overnight, their collective word had become law.

The oldest and most experienced of the three—both medically and politically—was sixty-year-old Nathaniel B. Emerson, who had been serving on the republic's Board of Health since his appointment by President Dole in 1896. The son of missionaries from New England, Emerson had been born on Oahu, where he grew up speaking Hawaiian among children in the village where his father served as pastor. He epitomized a rather amorphous group of second-generation whites known colloquially during the 1880s and 1890s as the "mission boys"—Americans who rose to positions of power and influence among the people their parents had come to convert to Christianity and capitalism.[1]

After Emerson completed school on Oahu with his Hawaiian friends, his parents sent him to Williams College in their native Massachusetts.

While he was a student, the Civil War broke out, and Emerson enlisted, along with many of his classmates, in a Massachusetts infantry regiment. Shrapnel from Confederate artillery fire tore his cap off during the Battle of Gettysburg in 1863, and he was wounded three times in the bloody spring offensive of 1864. Yet Emerson continued to fight with his regiment right through the surrender of Richmond in the spring of 1865. No one ever doubted either his mental determination or his physical courage.

Following discharge from the army, Emerson completed his baccalaureate at Williams and entered Harvard Medical School. After finishing his basic medical training in Boston, he transferred to the College of Physicians and Surgeons of New York City, in order to study surgery under Willard Parker. While in New York, Emerson also served as clinical assistant to O. Edouard Seguin, a national leader in the treatment of insanity. By the standards of that era, Emerson was thus working with individuals at the forefront of the medical profession. He received his MD degree in 1869 and developed a successful practice in New York City over the next decade. Interacting with the city's top physicians, he kept up to date on major medical developments throughout the United States and Europe, including the revolutionary field of bacteriology, which he enthusiastically embraced.

In 1878, S. G. Wilder, one of Emerson's boyhood friends from Oahu, became interior minister of the Kingdom of Hawaii. Wilder promptly wrote to Emerson, pleading with him to come back to the islands and help the government get leprosy under control. Emerson recognized that his old friend's plea was both medically and politically motivated, since the disfiguring disease not only ruined the lives of those afflicted but also threatened to tarnish Hawaii's reputation in the eyes of the rest of the world. Both white elites and Hawaiian aristocrats feared that no one would want to do business with them—much less voluntarily visit them—if their homeland was perceived as a dangerous string of leprous islands. The loyal mission boy agreed to tackle the task, closed his practice in New York City, and returned to the island of his birth as "general inspector of lepers and leper colonies." For the next twenty years, Emerson would remain more or less continuously active on the tumultuous and often perilous frontier between medicine and politics in Hawaii.[2]

As general inspector of lepers, Emerson toured the archipelago in search of concealed cases. The task of hunting down afflicted indigenous folk and wresting them from their families made him extremely unpopular with many ordinary Hawaiians and turned him into a symbol of medical imperialism. More than one family drew their guns on the doctor, but the

Civil War veteran unflinchingly worked to identify and remove everyone with an active case of leprosy to the leper colony at Kalaupapa, on a remote peninsula jutting out from the base of inaccessible cliffs on the island of Molokai. There, at least in theory, the afflicted could be treated by medical experts not available elsewhere; and whether their lives were improved or not, the lepers would at least be removed and isolated from the rest of the islands. Following his tour, Emerson went to the controversial Kalaupapa colony, which badly needed reorganization and upgrading. There he devoted himself so thoroughly to the well-being of his patients—some of whose relatives had previously threatened to shoot him—that they petitioned the government to keep him on as permanent supervisor.

With leprosy safely isolated on Molokai, Emerson moved in 1880 to Hawaii's next most sensitive medical post. He became "vaccinating officer" in Honolulu, where he was responsible for examining the health of incoming immigrants. The vast majority of the immigrants were Chinese and Japanese laborers, who were entering the islands from areas of the world that both white elites and Hawaiian aristocrats considered—even before the outbreak of bubonic plague—fonts of epidemic disease. Emerson served as medical gatekeeper, holding in quarantine anyone who appeared to be carrying a dangerous disease. He also routinely immunized all of the immigrants against smallpox, the one contagion against which medical doctors could then protect. For indigent people already in the city, Emerson opened and directed a new public dispensary, where health care was provided free of charge.

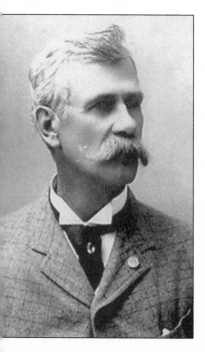

r. Nathaniel B. Emerson, senior member of the Honolulu Board of Health. lamiya Medical Heritage Center. awaii Medical Library

While working in Honolulu, Emerson met Dr. Sarah Eliza Peirce, who was practicing obstetrics and gynecology in the city. Like Emerson, Peirce had attended elementary school in Hawaii before going to New England in 1875 to study medicine. Since few regular medical schools in the United States at that time admitted women, Peirce enrolled at the Boston Homeopathic College, where she completed her medical degree in 1877. Also like Emerson, Peirce believed that the future of medicine lay not with homeopathy but with the new bacteriological sciences, so she went to Germany and France to learn about them before returning to Hawaii. Notwithstanding the thirteen-year gap in their ages, the two like-minded physicians married in 1885 and moved into a comfortable Victorian home on School Street, where they also maintained their medical offices.[3]

In 1887 Emerson found himself at the center of an especially nasty incident in the perennially tangled politics of public health in Hawaii. King David Kalakaua, who was often at odds with Hawaii's white elites during his tumultuous rule in the late 1880s, realized that many Hawaiians had long regarded European and American medical professionals like Emerson as agents of a way of life they disliked and distrusted. The king also understood that the officials responsible for the health of a society necessarily possessed—in addition to their legal authority—a great deal of cultural influence. Consequently, Kalakaua decided to try to override the Western-dominated Honolulu Board of Health, which determined medical policy throughout the kingdom. He proposed a new Hawaiian Board of Health, whose members the king intended to appoint himself. All members of the new board would be kahunas, or traditional Hawaiian healers, who would be granted an exclusive right to determine who could practice medicine in the islands. For Kalakaua, this was a symbolic effort to reassert indigenous authority over a society increasingly under the political influence and economic control of outsiders. To Western-trained doctors, the king's ploy seemed retrogressive and perverse. Christian missionaries, like Emerson's parents, saw the kahuna plan as an effort to revive pagan customs.[4]

Whites inside Kalakaua's badly fractured government blocked the king's efforts to shift legal licensing power to his kahunas and persuaded Emerson to take over as president of the original Honolulu Board of Health. After a two-month struggle that culminated in a showdown over keys to the agency's downtown office, the politically effective Emerson restored the supremacy of the Western-dominated board. In retaliation, an irate Hawaiian legislator introduced a bill to ban Emerson from practicing medicine in the islands. Though the bill was eventually defeated, Hawaiian members of the legislature managed to pass another law that banned the doctor from continuing in private practice while holding public medical posts.[5]

Following this confrontation in 1887, Emerson decided that the monarchical government he was theoretically serving could no longer be trusted with the long-term future of the islands. Like many of his friends, he convinced himself that the best future for Hawaii and Hawaiians lay under the protective custody of the United States, the nation he had once fought to preserve. In that conviction, he was hardly alone among the Western-trained doctors then practicing in Hawaii. Outraged and insulted that the king would seriously try to make them subservient to people they regarded as witch doctors, Honolulu's Western-trained physicians united in nearly unanimous and implacable opposition to indigenous rule. By attacking their professional status, Kalakaua had hit a sensitive spot. When the alliance of American planters and American merchants overthrew the Hawaiian monarchy in 1893, Hawaii's Western physicians were among the most ardent supporters of the coup.

Although his political experiences persuaded Emerson that the monarchy had become dysfunctional and dangerous, the mission-boy physician nonetheless retained his admiration for many aspects of the traditional Hawaiian culture. In 1893, even as he joined those Americans bent upon delivering the Hawaiian Islands to the United States, he presented a pioneering paper before the Hawaiian Historical Society that championed the extraordinary navigational prowess of the ancient Polynesians. At a time when few people were doing so, he continuously collected, translated, and preserved Hawaiian-language songs, chants, histories, legends, and epic tales. His collections were later given to the United States Bureau of American Ethnography and to the Huntington Library, where they remain among the most significant repositories of nineteenth-century Hawaiian-language works.[6]

Provided bacteriology retained its place of primacy, Emerson also remained reasonably tolerant of alternative methods of healing. Following their victory in the showdown with Kalakaua, for example, a group of Honolulu's Western-trained physicians approached the reempowered Board of Health with a demand to ban the importation of Japanese herbals. In its way, this proposal was as much an assertion of symbolic dominance as the king's kahuna scheme had been; in both cases the parties were trying to use control over public health care as a key component in the assertion of cultural authority. But Emerson bravely opposed the idea. "[I] am inclined to believe that [the herbals] had been of some benefit," the Board president told his colleagues, "and that certain of the patients seemed wedded to them." His arguments prevailed and importation continued.[7]

In sum, the senior member of the Board of Health was a complicated and somewhat paradoxical person. On the one hand, he was a scientifically progressive physician, trained by top figures in Western medicine and fully committed to the promise of bacteriology; on the other, he was realistic about what Western medicine could and could not do, and he remained tolerant of other approaches to healing. As a personal symbol of professional imperialism, Emerson had been targeted—literally and legislatively—by Hawaiians who hoped to reduce the power of outside whites; yet he nonetheless revered and preserved the Hawaiian traditions and Hawaiian language of his upbringing and became arguably the most important conservator of Hawaiian culture in his generation. Emerson's scholarly and religious mind-set coexisted somewhat incongruously but comfortably with an impressive record as a political infighter. No other physician in the islands had won more major victories on the battleground of Hawaiian public health than the battle-scarred war veteran Nathaniel Emerson.

Serving on the Board of Health with Emerson in the final years of the nineteenth century were a pair of longtime friends and medical partners, Francis R. Day and Clifford B. Wood. Forty-year-old Francis Day had been born in Missouri in 1859, then taken as an infant to Chicago when the Civil War broke out. His strongly pro-Union parents, upset with the political waffling of their border slave state and afraid for their own safety as ardent Free-Soilers, wanted to relocate to a securely pro-Union area. The family remained permanently in Chicago after the war, and Day went through public schools there before taking pre-medical training at the University of Michigan. In 1882 he graduated from the Chicago College of Physicians and Surgeons, then did an eighteen-month internship at Cook County Hospital, and headed to Europe for eight months of additional study. In Europe, he too embraced the new bacteriology.[8]

Day returned to Chicago, married the daughter of an older doctor in 1885, and was trying to establish a medical practice when his own health began to fail. Hoping to benefit from warmer climates and sea air, he signed on as a sort of circuit-riding ship's doctor for the Oceanic Steamship Company. When Day was only twenty-five, he and his bride headed for the South Pacific. On one of their voyages in 1886, the Days stopped at Honolulu, found the place enthralling, and decided to stay.

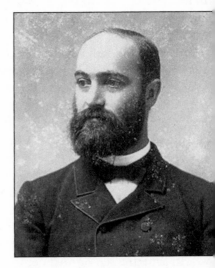

Dr. Francis R. Day, Honolulu Board of Health. Mamiya Medical Heritage Center. Hawaii Medical Library

Affable, outgoing, and erudite, Day quickly built a large practice among the white elites of his new city. Impressed with his solid scientific training and European polish, people found his medical manner immensely comforting and his personality unusually charming. He read both German and French fluently; he avidly practiced the rapidly advancing art of photography; and "a violin in his hands responded feelingly to the touch of a true musician," according to those who knew him. By all accounts, Day was the sort of man everyone in genteel Victorian society genuinely admired.

In accord with his most prominent patients and almost all of his professional colleagues, Day too came to strongly favor the annexation of Hawaii to his native United States. He was a leading member of the Hawaiian Society of the Sons of the American Revolution and an active participant in the secret Annexationist Club, which engineered the overthrow of Queen Liliuokalani. When the Honolulu Board of Health was reconstituted under the aegis of the new republic in 1894, President Dole's first appointment went to Day, his trusted medical confidant from the Annexationist Club. Day had been serving on the Board ever since, though he took a year off to return to Chicago and obtain another MD degree—from Rush Medical College, a more scientifically oriented and prestigious institution than the one he had graduated from ten years earlier. Day also doubled as chief port physician following the outbreak of the world plague epidemic. In that capacity his colleagues on the Honolulu Board of Health had sent him, at government expense, to China and Japan in 1897, to see firsthand how Asian ports were dealing with plague security.

The third physician on the Honolulu Board of Health in December 1899 was Day's medical partner and longtime friend, Clifford B. Wood. Wood's mother and father had been living in Cincinnati when he was born in 1859, but his father died when he was only a few months old, and his widowed mother returned to her own family in Chicago. From early childhood, Clifford's closest boyhood pal was his neighbor, Francis Day. Just four months apart in age, the two went in tandem through Chicago's public schools, the University of Michigan, and the Chicago College of Physicians and Surgeons. Following completion of medical school, they spent eighteen months interning together at Cook County Hospital before Day left for warmer climates.

Wood was doing staff work at Cook County and trying to build a private practice of his own when he began to receive letters from his old friend. Day extolled the tropical glories and professional opportunities he was finding in Honolulu, and he urged Wood to join him. Medicine was an extremely competitive business for a young doctor in Chicago at that time, another winter was coming on, and each one of Day's letters made Hawaii sound more appealing than the last. So Wood decided in the fall of 1886 to follow his friend to Honolulu. As persuasive as he was resolute, Wood convinced a young nurse at Cook County—"over the strenuous objections of her parents"—to come with him. The two were formally married in a ceremony at the Days' house in Honolulu the following year.

Once in Hawaii, Wood joined Day's circle of influential Americans. He too became an active member of the Sons of the American Revolution and of the camera club. Those ties, in turn, helped him secure a series of public health appointments. Following a short stint as a district physician outside the city, Wood returned to Honolulu as official city physician. The $2,400 salary for that job was too low to support the lifestyle he wanted, so he resigned to concentrate on his private practice. Even so, Wood had remained active in public health affairs through the early 1890s, serving variously as director of the public dispensary that Emerson once ran, surgeon to the Kakaako Hospital for quarantined immigrants, police department doctor, and physician to the Lunalilo home, which cared for indigent Hawaiians. He also inspected and vaccinated children in the public schools and became what would now be called chief of surgery at Queens Hospital.

Like his colleagues, Wood became an avid proponent of American annexation during the late 1880s. When the coup against Liliuokalani took place in 1893, Wood served prominently in the Citizens' Guard, the annexationists' paramilitary arm. From the leg of a Hawaiian policeman, Wood extracted the only bullet that hit anyone during the coup and kept it on his desk as a souvenir of what he considered a glorious event. Shortly after proclaiming the Republic of Hawaii, President Dole appointed Wood to join his friend Day on the Board of Health. In 1895 Wood was also elected to a term on the Council of State, which made him simultaneously a member of the government's highest decision-making body, a ranking officer in that government's military organization, and a member of the government's Board of Health. Wood's many over-

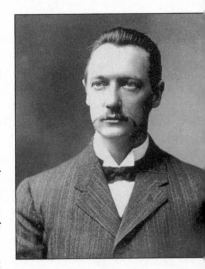

Dr. Clifford B. Wood, Honolulu Board of Health. Mamiya Medical Heritage Center. Hawaii Medical Library

lapping posts clearly illustrated the interlocking roles played by the American elites in Hawaii during the late 1890s, and lent credibility to the opinion of Chinatown residents that the Board of Health was simply the not-to-be-trusted Dole regime in another guise.

Like Day, Wood had also visited China and Japan at government expense to investigate health matters for himself. During a three-month tour in 1896, he gathered what information he could, especially about the plague epidemic, then returned and presented a paper before the Hawaiian Medical Association summarizing what he had learned. After seeing health conditions in Asia, he was even more convinced that Hawaii should cast its lot with the United States. "The only politics I have is annexation," he declared famously at that time, and he repeated that statement often in the ensuing three years. When Wood's wife gave birth to their third child in September 1899, the couple named the boy Sanford Ballard Dole Wood.[9]

In the spring of 1899, Day and Wood had merged their separate private practices into a single professional partnership, which they were operating from an office in Beretania Street when the outbreak of plague in Chinatown propelled them to positions of unprecedented power. Along with their senior colleague on the Board of Health, they found themselves part of a triumvirate running America's most recent acquisition. In additional to their personal friendships and associations, the three physicians on the Board of Health in 1899 had two other overriding things in common that bound them together: their commitment to bacteriology in the service of public health and their commitment to the goals of the administration that appointed them. Particularly in the latter, they were truly the government's plague fighters.

Three laymen also served formally on the republic's Board of Health. One was Henry E. Cooper, then Hawaii's attorney general and the elected officer to whom the Board officially reported. He was on the Board because the constitution of the republic stipulated that the attorney general would function automatically as titular president of the Board of Health. The other two were George W. Smith and L. D. Keliipio. Smith, a prominent representative of the American commercial elites, had been appointed earlier in 1899; Keliipio had served for three years, but he had seldom been active in the Board's affairs, and little is known about him. As a practical matter, the three civilians attended the Board's daily meetings only sporadically and deferred to the three physicians on all matters of public policy.[10]

Though not formally appointed to the Board, a fourth physician, Duncan A. Carmichael, acted as an ex-officio advisor to the medical triumvirate of

Emerson, Day, and Wood. Carmichael had been born in Montreal, Canada, in 1851 and received his MD degree from McGill University in 1873, before emigrating to the United States. In 1881 he joined the United States Marine Hospital Service, the rapidly expanding nineteenth-century predecessor of the United States Public Health Service. Well regarded inside the Marine Hospital Service, the expatriate Canadian doctor had steadily advanced from post to post; he was now at midcareer and appeared to be on the fast track.

When the Hawaiian annexation resolution passed Congress in 1898, the Marine Hospital Service sent Carmichael to Honolulu as their first superintendent of operations there. The assignment represented a significant boost for Carmichael, since the newly created Pacific post was located in an attractive place and was a highly visible job under the circumstances. Carmichael had primary responsibility for insuring that American soldiers and sailors fighting in the Philippines could count on healthful conditions when passing back and forth through Hawaii. In his first year, Carmichael successfully persuaded his federal agency to pay for two additional hospitals in America's newest possession, and they were promptly built under his direction, one in Honolulu and one in Hilo.

Carmichael and the three physicians on the Honolulu Board of Health became trusted friends and like-minded, science-oriented colleagues almost immediately. This was fortunate, since their formal lines of authority were hopelessly blurred under the "existing government" rules and they might easily have become professional rivals instead. Who could say, for example, where the continuing health responsibilities of the Dole regime ended and

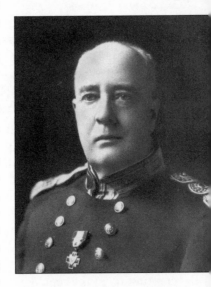

Dr. Duncan A. Carmichael in his Public Health Service uniform. National Library of Medicine

the legitimate health concerns of the United States government with regard to its military personnel and its newly acquired subjects began? But Carmichael and the three Board physicians had the same goal—to keep the islands safe from disease—and they made the same basic bacteriological assumption about contagious epidemics—that the health of every resident impacted that of everyone else. Consequently, Carmichael allowed his friends on the Honolulu Board direct access to the latest medical communications available through the Marine Hospital Service, and he shared federal medical supplies with the Board's physicians, on the rationale of keeping Honolulu safe for American military personnel.[11]

Carmichael and the Board's three medical members also shared a strong belief that the future of public health lay with bacteriology. So did Carmichael's federal agency back in Washington, D.C. During the late summer and early fall of 1899, shortly before plague appeared in Chinatown, the Marine Hospital Service had moved beyond drawings of *pestis* and distributed actual slides of the bacterium to U.S. government physicians stationed around the world, including Carmichael in Honolulu. Carmichael shared the slides with his friends on Dole's Board of Health. Those slides became the norm against which Hoffman, the city bacteriologist, would test for plague.[12]

On a personal level, Carmichael had found his new assignment thoroughly delightful. He liked to hike in the islands, he rediscovered ancient Hawaiian caves near Koko Head, and he brought to light a number of lost petroglyphs. Honolulu's white elites made the physician from the Marine Hospital Service feel at home—no wonder, since he was the first civilian representative of the government they had been so eager to welcome into the islands. In the summer of 1899, the forty-eight-year-old widower married Alice McKee Hastings, a wealthy Honolulu widow, following a whirlwind, high-society courtship. If the new Mrs. Carmichael's reputation as a tempestuous and difficult personality cast any shadows into the future, Carmichael himself did not see them. Until the winter of 1899, his life in Honolulu could hardly have been more congenial, either professionally or personally. With the appearance of bubonic plague, however, his responsibilities increased sharply, and in his capacity as unofficial counselor to the three physicians in charge, he would find himself working under intensely strained conditions for the next five months.[13]

The events of December 12 also propelled a fifth physician from relative obscurity into the public spotlight. That man was the city's bacteriologist, Walter Hoffman, whom Herbert summoned to help with the first autopsy at the Wing Wo Tai Company. Just twenty-seven years old, Hoffman had graduated from medical school in his native Germany less than two years earlier. Landing in Honolulu as ship's doctor for a boatload of Austrian immigrants, Hoffman liked the city so much that he applied for a license to practice medicine there. In the course of examining his application, the three physicians on the Board of Health noticed that Hoffman had taken advanced training in the latest bacteriological techniques, first in Berlin and then briefly at the Johns Hopkins Medical School. They granted him a license at the end of 1898 and kept their eyes on the young newcomer.[14]

Hoffman had grown up amid the intellectual aristocracy of Berlin, where his father was a professor. Socially adept and fully at home in the worlds of art and music, the well-bred young German with the flashing red whiskers and the gilt-edged credentials quickly made an impression among Honolulu's white elites. For Emerson, Day, and Wood, that impression was altogether positive. They marveled at Hoffman's skills with a microscope, all the more remarkable since a collegiate fencing accident had blinded him in one eye. Remembering the flap that had forced their predecessors in 1895 to send cholera samples to mainland laboratories, the Board's three physicians determined to take advantage of Hoffman's fortuitous appearance in Honolulu. In August 1899 they created the new post of city bacteriologist and persuaded Hoffman to accept the job.

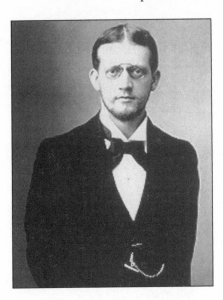

Dr. Walter Hoffman, Honolulu city bacteriologist. Mamiya Medical Heritage Center. Hawaii Medical Library

Hoffman made a less positive impression on some of the city's other white physicians. Most of the skeptics were older doctors who had practiced pre-bacteriological medicine for many years in the islands. They resented this continental aristocrat as an upstart competitor putting on airs, a come-lately neophyte who was a bit too up-to-date for his own good. In their view, the new city bacteriologist knew little or nothing about health matters in Hawaii, and they thought of him in the same way they thought of the bacteriology he practiced: as untried and untested. They said little while Hoffman spent his time examining the Honolulu water supply, but they would eventually bring heavy pressure on the young outsider when the arrival of plague suddenly and dramatically changed the face of medical politics.

In many ways, the medical team directing the battle against plague and running the Hawaiian Islands looked impressive. In command was a triumvirate that included a skillful veteran (Emerson) and two capable physicians in their professional prime, one of whom was unusually well regarded (Day), while the other was decisive, persuasive, and administratively able (Wood). Those three were supported, in turn, by a fully cooperative United States public health officer tagged for the fast track (Carmichael), and a medical bacteriologist splendidly trained in the latest techniques of that new science (Hoffman). From other perspectives, however, the same team could look quite different. The ruling triumvirate could be characterized as a battle-weary physician with plenty of public scars (Emerson), plus two boyhood pals from Chicago (Day and Wood), who had somehow gotten each other in over their heads after being appointed by political cronies. Those three were supported, in turn, by a United States public health officer who was unsure about his own authority under the "existing government" (Carmichael), and a recently arrived outsider whose one-eyed bacteriological investigations were resented by many of Honolulu's longtime practitioners. Both views were freely expressed on the streets of the city.

5

Quarantine

"P LAGUE IS IN THE CITY" announced the headlines of Honolulu's English-language newspapers on December 13, the morning after Dole's "existing government" turned the Hawaiian Islands over to the Honolulu Board of Health. Hawaiian, Japanese, and Chinese publications did the same in their own languages. "BOARD OF HEALTH IN CHARGE," confirmed other front-page stories. And along with pleas for calm came requests for citizen involvement in the emergency efforts already planned for the days ahead: "VOLUNTEER HEALTH INSPECTORS PLEASE REPORT AT THE BOARD OF HEALTH IMMEDIATELY." Though held at bay for five years, the world pandemic had finally breached the city's defenses. Honolulu mobilized a counterattack in less than forty-eight hours.

Despite repeated reminders that this epidemic had rarely attacked Caucasians elsewhere in the world, observers immediately noticed that the headlines of December 13 were generating more intense anxieties among Honolulu's white residents than any previous health threat ever had. "On every hand were signs of extreme public tension," reported the *Pacific Commercial Advertiser* that morning, "and these were increased by the characteristic Honolulu rumors." One editor even hypothesized that people of European descent might have inherited an abnormally intense fear of plague from their ancestors' catastrophic experiences in the Middle Ages.[1]

More likely sources of distress among Honolulu's whites were their deeply held cultural assumptions that linked the presence of plague to "diseased" social and political ways of life. Plague had long been among the most powerful metaphors in Western consciousness, a negative marker that went back even further than Biblical imagery. Consequently, while the city's whites did not anticipate sudden waves of widespread death among themselves, they were terrified, as the press recognized plainly, that observers around the world might begin to associate their city not with plague-free northern Europe and the New World, but with such debased urban centers as Bombay, where plague was still "slaughtering three hundred victims *per diem*," or Hong Kong, where plague had lingered continuously for the "past two hundred years." Where order and hygiene prevailed, plague could be resisted; where chaos and filth reigned, plague could establish itself. So if the epidemic now gained a foothold in the city, Honolulu faced the prospect of appearing to be, or perhaps even becoming, "Asian."[2]

Sensing the dismay of whites—not to mention a genuine fear for their lives among Asian residents—all of the English-language dailies cautioned against panic and urged full support for the Board of Health. "Encouragement may be drawn from our experience in the cholera epidemic," stated the *Hawaiian Gazette*. "So brethren, be of good cheer. The bubonic plague, though undeniably with us, is not likely to plague us long . . . and it is but a matter of a few days before the active and intelligent labors of the Board of Health ought to bring the city out of its trouble and permit the inhabitants, white, yellow and brown, to resume their unruffled courses." The *Advertiser* repeated the same admonitions. "Stand by the leaders," urged the *Evening Bulletin*, because "next to the plague itself a general stampede caused by fear" now posed the city's greatest danger. Even the *Independent*, which for years had bluntly castigated virtually every policy initiated by what it alternately called the "the Dole gang" or "Hawaii's puppet regime," now rallied strongly behind the government's resolve to contain and destroy the invading epidemic.[3]

Responding to the intense medical and sociopolitical pressures on them, Emerson, Day, and Wood quickly implemented the policies they had hastily agreed upon the day after You Chong and the four others perished. Hoping to prevent the disease from spreading beyond Oahu, the physicians ordered an immediate halt to all inter-island shipping in the Hawaiian archipelago. Should plague reach the other islands, they feared widespread death among Asian plantation workers and a probable collapse of Hawaii's economy. Despite a mad rush of captains to weigh anchor before the order went into effect, only one boat managed to get out of the harbor.[4]

On Oahu itself, the Board members imposed travel restrictions in and out of Honolulu. They were quite rightly afraid that people might try to escape the threat of plague in the city, as urban populations had done elsewhere for centuries and as some residents were already doing in Honolulu, and thereby inadvertently spread the disease to neighboring plantations on their own island. Reflecting the internationally held opinion that Asian races were more susceptible to bubonic plague than other races, and hence more likely to be its carriers, both the inter-island ban and the Honolulu city ban were absolute for Chinese and Japanese residents. Non-Asians could apply for special travel exceptions if they were willing to submit to medical examinations by Board-appointed physicians. The U.S. Army physician at Camp McKinley, which had recently been established several miles from downtown Honolulu on the leeward slope of Diamond Head, expressed "little doubt about the diagnosis" of plague and forbade American troops from entering the city.[5]

Within Honolulu, the three physicians also imposed the policy that Chinatown residents had been hoping to avoid: an intra-city quarantine of that district. No one could come or go from that area without permission from a Board-appointed agent. To enforce the quarantine, Emerson, Day, and Wood called out the Dole government's national guard. Though physicians carefully explained the health risks of quarantine duty to the guardsmen, every member of the force volunteered to serve. The paramilitary guardsmen, many of whom were Hawaiians, were immediately deployed around the perimeter of the district, with their largest numbers concentrated along Nuuanu Street, which marked the unofficial border between Chinatown and the city's Euro-American commercial center immediately to the east.

By sealing off the district where all the early deaths had occurred, the physicians on the Board of Health hoped to isolate the epidemic. Underlying this policy was a profoundly spatial, almost geographical, understanding of epidemic disease that went back at least to the Middle Ages. Plague in particular had long been thought to exist in defined spaces; it seemed to invade, entrench, and occupy particular areas very like an alien army might establish zones of occupation. Wood stated the Board's belief succinctly: "plague is preeminently a disease of locality and place." By sealing off the infected areas, he and his colleagues hoped to prevent the enemy from establishing any new zones of occupation or enlarging the one already under attack.[6]

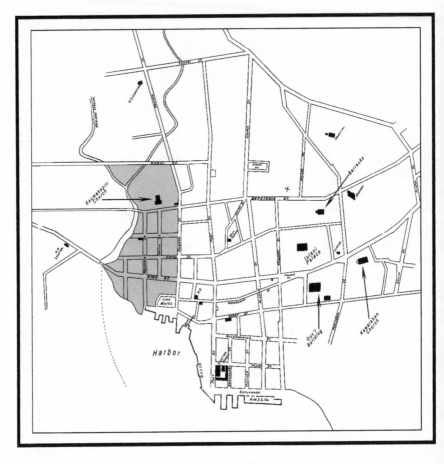

Central Honolulu, with quarantined area shaded.

Modern bacteriology meshed perfectly with those long-standing assumptions and provided a scientific rationale for continuing to impose quarantines against bubonic plague. The enemy now had a face and a name, and each *pestis* bacterium could easily be thought of as a tiny hostile soldier who had to get physically from place to place in order to do any damage. By stopping the bacteria's most likely modes of conveyance, public health officials hoped to trap them in confined areas. Measures could then be taken inside those quarantined areas to destroy the bacteria, either directly or by eliminating the conditions they needed to survive.

The area placed under quarantine formed an uneven rectangle extending inland from Honolulu's commercial waterfront. The other three sides were bounded by Nuuanu Street on the east, Kukui Street and a strip of undeveloped land on the north, and a small stream to the west. Shoulder-to-shoulder wooden buildings predominated throughout the densely built district. The vast majority of the buildings were two-story structures facing on streets or alleys, although some buildings had an extra half-story or full story added above the standard two. Wedged behind and between most of the permanent buildings were hundreds of shacks, lean-tos, and storage sheds of irregular sizes and shapes. All of the latter had been erected in flagrant disregard of the city's health and building codes. With a few notable exceptions, living conditions in Chinatown were generally squalid. Residents typically lived in the same building where they worked, or in adjoining, often interconnecting and somewhat mazelike rooming houses, where scores of single men typically shared extremely tight quarters.[7]

Even before the outbreak of plague, Chinatown was regarded as Honolulu's worst slum and as a generally unhealthy area. It received only a meager flow of fresh water from the hills above the city, yet parts of Chinatown near sea level remained mucky and stagnant year around. Sanitary inspections by the Board of Health would reveal overflowing cesspools, privies disgorging their contents, garbage rotting almost everywhere, and alleys impassable due to large piles of refuse. As the plague emergency played itself out, angry debates took place over who bore responsibility for those conditions—residents, owners, on-site property managers, absentee landlords, or the Board of Health itself for not enforcing its own sanitary laws in that part of the city.[8]

Observers generally believed that about 5,000 people were crammed into Chinatown at any given time, though some members of the Board of Health initially feared there might be twice that number. Contrary to its name, not all of the people who lived in Chinatown were Chinese, nor did all of the Chinese in Honolulu live in Chinatown. Roughly 3,000 of the city's approximately 10,000 Chinese residents lived there. The rest were scattered around Honolulu in smaller Asian neighborhoods or in accommodations provided by their employers. According to a survey done three years earlier, the area that found itself under quarantine contained 72 of Honolulu's 153 Chinese stores.[9]

Economic disparities inside Chinatown were extreme. At the top were a handful of powerful merchants, manufacturers, and investment managers who wielded tremendous influence in the community, though not all of them actually lived there. Five years earlier, those leaders had mobilized their countrymen to successfully resist discriminatory measures proposed against Asians, but they were powerless under the present circumstances to stop the emergency plague quarantine. And since a prolonged quarantine would badly hurt their Chinatown businesses, they had a strong incentive to cooperate—within reason—with the Board of Health and get it over with.

The powerful Chinese merchant class was linked to a small cadre of professionals, newspaper editors, and law clerks. Most of the law clerks represented Chinese interests in white law offices. At the bottom of Chinatown's hierarchy were day laborers who toiled at menial jobs throughout the city. Many of them unmarried men living in Honolulu on their own, they worked as stevedores for the city's immediately adjacent wharves, house servants for the city's wealthy residents, groomsmen for the city's stables, and laborers for the light manufacturing and merchant firms owned and operated by more successful Chinese. Several hundred Chinese "floaters" without regular employment of any sort were essentially vagrant, working and sleeping throughout Chinatown wherever an opportunity presented itself.[10]

Chinatown's middle class consisted of budding entrepreneurs and skilled tradesmen. Some were trusted employees in white businesses; others were involved in the city's booming construction projects; a few bought and sold items of all sorts in the surrounding countryside. Among those upwardly striving residents in 1899 was Chung Kun Ai. At the age of fourteen, Chung had emigrated to Hawaii from south China with his father, who worked in the coffee trade. Chung was left with friends in Honolulu, where his father was persuaded to enroll him as one of only 4 Chinese children among 108 students at the prominent Bishop School. One of Chung's classmates and best friends at the school was Sun Tai Cheong, the same person who became a classmate of Li and Kong when he returned to China for his medical degree and emerged as Dr. Sun Yat-Sen. Chung remained a steadfast supporter of Sun and helped host the famous revolutionary during his many trips back to Hawaii in later years.[11]

After failing in a tailoring partnership, Chung spent eleven years as the principal business manager of a vast ranching empire on the island of Hawaii owned by a prominent white planter, James I. Dowsett. That post gave Chung valuable mercantile experience and earned him the trust and respect of many European and American businessmen. Following Dowsett's death in 1898, Chung struck out on his own. With the help of a Hawaiian friend, Chung leased land in lower Chinatown immediately adjacent to the harbor. There he launched City Mill, an enterprise designed to process rice and lumber. With the backing of both white and Chinese investors, he amassed enough capital to purchase steam-driven equipment and hire laborers. By December 1899, the lumber portion of the business, which could be done outdoors, was vigorously underway, and City Mill's impressive new building was almost completed.[12]

Since the Republic of Hawaii barred all Chinese from citizenship, the Chinese residents of Hawaii remained—at least in theory—subjects of the Qing Empire back in China, even if they had been in the islands for two or three generations. Nominally, therefore, their interests were represented by the empire's officially appointed consul to Hawaii, Yang Wei Pin, who was formally recognized by the Dole government. But Consul Yang spent most of his time and official leverage looking out only for Honolulu's leading Chinese businessmen, especially those involved in trade with China itself. Critics openly assailed Yang as biased and corrupt. Yang's own vice-consul, the well-respected Gu Kim Fui, who had led the drive to build a Chinese hospital, intimated years later that the Qing consul favored those who had sufficient money and enough finesse to find ways of paying him under the table.[13]

While the Chinese residents of Chinatown generally tried to present a united front to the outside world, they differed sharply among themselves, mostly over the future of their ancient homeland. Some of the Chinese who disparaged ambassador Yang no doubt did so because they, like Li and Kong, opposed the absolute monarchy he represented. They favored

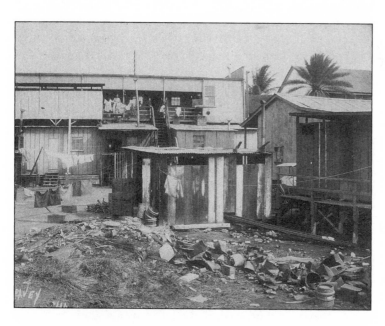

A backyard in Chinatown. Hawaii State Archives

a shift to some form of constitutional monarchy back home, or to a modified parliamentary system similar to those that existed in Europe at the time. Still others inside Chinatown believed that the Qing Empire was not worth preserving in any form. This group favored thoroughgoing revolution, though they differed among themselves over what postrevolutionary China might look like. The Qing government regularly posted bounties on the heads of those known to be openly advocating revolution, but the Chinese in Honolulu stopped short of turning one another over to rival agents. The various factions did, however, regularly issue handbills, sometimes refuse to do business with one another, and overtly shun their opponents socially—as Li and Kong had found out in the weeks leading up to the quarantine.[14]

Close to fifteen hundred of Chinatown's residents under quarantine in December 1899—almost a third—were Japanese. The vast majority of the city's Japanese residents had come to Hawaii quite recently, after white sugar planters stopped importing Chinese laborers and stepped up their recruitment of Japanese laborers. As a result, the Japanese population in the archipelago as a whole had roughly tripled just since 1896; during 1899, with Japanese immigration at an all-time high, the Japanese had suddenly emerged as the largest ethnic group on the islands. Lorrin Thurston had used the exploding numbers of Japanese in Hawaii as one of his arguments for American annexation: if the United States did not act quickly, he warned, then Japan, having just won Formosa in the first Sino-Japanese War (1894–95), might decide to claim the Hawaiian archipelago next. Japanese naval vessels had played games of bluff with American naval vessels off Honolulu harbor on the eve of the annexation, when the Dole administration challenged the imperial Japanese government's direct control over the flow of Japanese workers.[15]

Against that tense background, the Japanese presence in the city had recently become quite formidable. Their total numbers in the city were estimated to be about seven thousand, which meant that less than a quarter of the city's Japanese residents lived in Chinatown—a smaller percentage than Honolulu's Chinese. But in economic terms, Chinatown was even more important to the Japanese community as a whole than it was to the Chinese community, since most of the city's major Japanese businesses were located there. Several of them, especially the ones engaged in large-scale trade with Japan, were rapidly overtaking their white counterparts.[16]

While most of the Chinese in Chinatown lived in the lower part of the district close to the harbor, most of the Japanese living in the quarantined zone resided in the more recently developed upper part of the district, away from the waterfront. Overwhelmingly single males, the Japanese of Chinatown worked in light manufacturing, heavy labor, construction trades, restaurants, stables, and a host of service jobs from gardening to retail clerking. Many of them were packed into miserable boardinghouses in upper Chinatown while they waited for plantation assignments on the outer islands. Collectively the Japanese who lived in Chinatown comprised the lowest socioeconomic tier of Honolulu's Japanese residents. Even the editor of the Japanese-language newspaper *Hawaii Shimpo*, whose publishing facilities were located in Chinatown, remembered Japanese living conditions in Chinatown at the time of the plague as "unimaginably unsanitary."[17]

Representing the Japanese residents of Hawaii was the imperial Japanese ambassador, Saito Miki, whom the Dole government had formally recognized as consul-general in September 1898. Extensive correspondence files in the Hawaiian state archives suggest that Consul Saito took seriously his charge to promote the welfare of all his countrymen in Hawaii, not just his business associates. The Dole administration, in turn, respected Saito and considered him effective. Along with the ambassador, at the top of Honolulu's Japanese community were successful retail merchants, import and export dealers, labor brokers, newspaper editors, light manufacturers, and professionals. Among the last category were at least a dozen Japanese physicians trained in Western medicine. Saito and the other leaders of the Japanese community commanded the respect of most Japanese residents, but had ongoing trouble dealing with a number of unsavory brothel keepers, gamblers, and organized crime figures among their countrymen.[18]

The third major group of Chinatown residents who found themselves confined together under quarantine was made up of nearly 1,000 Hawaiians. Most of the Hawaiians in Chinatown were relatively poor in comparison with the approximately 12,000 Hawaiians living elsewhere around Honolulu, but some of the Hawaiians in Chinatown, particularly the most elderly, were there because they wanted to remain in homes their families had occupied for generations before the influx of Asians. Many of the district's Hawaiians left Chinatown each morning for jobs in the city center or on the wharves. Several also left to fish, returning each evening with fresh food for their families and neighbors.[19]

The symbolic center of the traditional Hawaiian community in Chinatown—and the symbolic center for most Hawaiian Christians throughout the city—was Kaumakapili Church on Beretania Street. Its congregation had originally been organized to serve converted Hawaiian commoners, since the older Kawaiahao congregation, with its church near the Iolani Palace, had catered to the Hawaiian aristocracy. Ordinary Hawaiians still came from all over the city to worship every Sunday at Kaumakapili. While a struggling young lawyer, Sanford Dole had taught Sunday school there. The church's magnificent twin spires, the tallest in the city, dominated Honolulu's western skyline and appeared even taller than they were because the church sat upon the brow of a gentle ridge above the center of Chinatown. Those spires were easily visible from almost any vantage point in the region. The many Japanese who had recently moved in around Kaumakapili also admired what they fondly called—using the old term for Hawaiians—"the Kanaka Temple."[20]

Chinatown also sheltered small numbers of other people of other ethnicities. A few score Portuguese lived in the quarantined district, as did semitransient sailors who hailed from places as distant from one another as Spain and the East Indies. Several non-Hawaiian Polynesians who had migrated to Honolulu from places like Samoa and Tonga had found refuge in Chinatown, and a handful of people from Micronesia also lived there. One of the district's first five plague victims, whose deaths had triggered the health emergency and quarantine in the first place, was a twenty-four-year-old man from the Gilbert Islands, now the Republic of Kiribati, named Nakauaila. He had come over two thousand miles to seek his fortune in the bustling mid-Pacific port of Honolulu, only to have a desperately choking rat flea inject him with a deadly dose of bubonic plague.[21]

To monitor the situation inside the quarantined zone, the Board of Health called for physicians and other qualified volunteers to conduct daily (later twice-daily) house-to-house inspections. Each inspector or team of inspectors was responsible for a specific subdistrict. Any suspicious illnesses and all deaths had to be reported immediately. Patients with suspicious illnesses would be removed to special quarantine hospitals for observation. The Board of Health promised that a representative would be available in the office for consultation at any time of the day or night. With these measures, Emerson, Day and Wood hoped to stay abreast of developments as they unfolded.

Under the terms of the quarantine, no one residing inside Chinatown on December 12 was allowed out until further notice. National guardsmen patrolled the official perimeter around the clock. Lines were painted down the middle of boundary streets to prevent people from intermingling on the periphery of the quarantined zone. Still, people managed to slip out of Chinatown, particularly at night, and melt into Asian and Hawaiian communities in other parts of the city, often joining friends or relatives. As Wood later acknowledged, "it was no easy matter to keep 8,000 or 10,000 people confined to a small district in the heart of town, when many of them wanted nothing more than to get out. There were, undoubtedly, many escapes."[22]

The perimeters of the quarantined district were perhaps more permeable from the outside than from the inside. The volunteer medical inspectors, for example, came and went daily. National guardsmen who had direct contact with the quarantined population relaxed at public theaters throughout the city when off duty. Various contractors and work crews received passes to take excavating machines and cleanup equipment into the quarantined district; then they hauled out wagon loads of material for disposal elsewhere and returned to their homes outside Chinatown at night. Security was lax. A stack of access passes was stolen from one of the guard huts. Both the Chinese and Japanese consuls were allowed to visit regularly and observe conditions within the supposedly isolated zone.[23]

Though far from perfect, the quarantine nonetheless imposed genuine hardships almost from beginning. Idle workers trapped inside the quarantined area were reported to be gambling and fighting. Because their printing facilities were inside the area, most of the city's non–English language newspapers were forced to cease publication, since they could not distribute their papers to their subscribers, most of whom lived outside Chinatown. Foodstuffs like meat and fish spoiled quickly in the tropical climate and could not be replaced. Unable to get out to fish, Hawaiians in particular felt the shortages. Opposition English-language newspapers reminded "the military government established in Honolulu" that they were still "servants of the public" and had a responsibility to provide for the "men, women, and children starving in the quarantined district under the military rule." Private relief organizations formed outside the quarantined district and negotiated ways to get food, including several tons of poi, into the sealed-off area.[24]

Chinatown residents considered the regime of daily inspections to be the most intrusive and personally objectionable of the Board's antiplague initiatives. Intimate bodily inspection by strangers seemed insulting, unnecessary, and ineffectual. Partly to end the need for the regular inspections, some Chinatown residents heeded the pleas of their business leaders and actively cooperated with the Board's efforts to clean and disinfect the district. Volunteer crews from inside the area worked with authorized crews from outside to remove garbage and to empty privies, even though the outside crews were being paid by the Board of Health and the crews from inside Chinatown were not being paid at all—yet another way in which

Chinatown's residents felt discriminated against. Even so, white inspectors optimistically reported that many district residents were helping with the cleanup "willingly, as they [were] anxious to break the quarantine and be at liberty once more."[25]

Not everyone pitched in. Handbills posted in the quarantined area openly attacked the Chinese consul and vice-consul as "worse than useless" when it came to looking out for the welfare of ordinary residents. Other posters made overt death threats against the Qing representatives, who were accused of caring more about trade goods than people. For his cooperation with Emerson, Day, and Wood, and for his outspoken support of the Board's policies, Li Khai Fai was assaulted by a hostile crowd inside the quarantined zone and barely escaped by dashing off on his bicycle. Protesters also castigated Tong San Kai, the hospital director who had assisted the Board's physicians in their investigations of the first five deaths.[26]

The confinement of so many Asian workers in Chinatown, in the words of a white paper, also had "a somewhat depressing effect on the commercial affairs of their Caucasian neighbors." Though the Chinese consul and vice-consul protested the closing of Chinatown's businesses when white businesses were allowed to remain open in the rest of the city, the quarantine resulted in a citywide slowdown. The Chamber of Commerce asked the Board of Health to consider establishing smaller quarantine zones outside Chinatown, where workers could be housed under observation for a safe period of time and then return to their jobs, but the physicians refused. Elsewhere in the city, the Board members suspended school indefinitely, and most restaurants closed, many from lack of workers. The quarantine's terms severely curtailed all forms of public transportation. Shipping came almost to a halt, as incoming goods had to be isolated and fumigated, and most of the men who usually worked on the wharves were confined in Chinatown, just across the street from where they would ordinarily be loading and unloading ships.[27]

Hawaiians visiting in Honolulu from other islands found themselves forbidden to return home without special passes from the Board. The Hawaiian-language press condemned the Board not for its "efforts to [defeat] the black fever—if it is, in fact, the black fever," but for its "crookedness" in the enforcement of its own rules, since whites found the travel passes easier to obtain than Hawaiians did. *Ke Aloha Aina* also called for legal action to be taken against Board of Health agents alleged to be selling inter-island travel passes under false pretenses, and the Hawaiians protested against the liberties allowed to those whose "money makes them immune from the grip of bubonic plague." Hawaiians also suspected that "the doctors of the Board of Health" had caught the "bubonic-plague-like disease of greed" from their friends in the Dole administration, accusing them of erecting the quarantine barriers "so that white [businesses] can profit."[28]

To support their accusations of racial bias, the Chinese pointed out that the quarantine line had been drawn to include Chung Kun Ai's brand-new City Mill, which fronted on the harbor, but excluded the white-owned Honolulu Iron Works—Honolulu's largest industry—whose grounds were immediately contiguous to City Mill. The protesters certainly had a point: on the quarantine maps, the Honolulu Iron Works property appeared as a small peninsula extending from the white commercial district along the waterfront into lower Chinatown. Moreover, rumors circulated that employees of the Iron Works who lived inside Chinatown were being allowed to cross the quarantine line and continue working regular shifts as long as they did not venture beyond the foundry's grounds. Consul Yang also identified a Chinese store on the other side of the Iron Works that appeared to be as arbitrarily inside the line as the Iron Works were artificially outside it and a Chinese-occupied block along Nuuanu Street that might logically have been excluded from the quarantine zone.[29]

Some Japanese businessmen believed that the abruptly declared quarantine was actually directed at them, not the Chinese. They suspected that the emergency policy was just another thinly disguised effort by white businessmen in the annexationist camp to find ways of curtailing the rapidly escalating economic power of their Japanese competitors. To minimize the impact of the quarantine on their businesses, Japanese merchants actively smuggled goods in and out of the quarantined zone. Whenever detected, Wood reported, the Japanese merchants "simply laughed and treated the [Board's regulations] as a joke."[30]

Under their emergency edicts, Emerson, Day, and Wood also assumed complete authority over the disposal of the dead. Bodies from anywhere in the city had to be inspected personally by Hoffman, who would take tissue samples for microscopic examination. If he found evidence of the *pestis* bacillus, the remains would be cremated as quickly as possible. Behind this policy lay a fear that plague bacteria might somehow escape from a buried corpse and survive in soil or in groundwater to attack again. Such fears were widely held by public health officials around the world and probably originated with Yersin and Kitasato themselves, both of whom had previously studied agronomy and therefore knew that soils harbored many different sorts of bacteria. Yersin claimed to find *pestis* as deep as eighteen inches below the surface of the ground during the outbreak in Hong Kong. Kitasato, who was conducting Japan's battle against the world epidemic, insisted that plague sites remain under quarantine for a full year, in order to make certain that the ground was completely decontaminated.[31]

Though Emerson, Day, and Wood regarded the cremation of plague victims as scientifically logical, their order alienated many Chinese. In an effort to sustain the tradition of burying the dead in their ancestral lands, many overseas Chinese practiced a system whereby they interred the dead for some years wherever they died, then had their bones disinterred and sent back to China. Cremation not only rendered that impossible, but also raised the specter of spiritual oblivion. British orders to cremate plague victims in Hong Kong had provoked rioting in 1894. The government plague fighters failed to explain the rationale behind their cremation edict to the Chinese, and the white press fanned already tense race relations by applauding the procedures not only as a prudent health measure but also as a demonstration "to a number of the prejudiced nationalities" that cremation was "an excellent manner in which to dispose of the dead."[32]

Following "the fashion set in the cholera epidemic" five years before, as well as the international protocols agreed upon in Europe, the three physicians launched another immediate and massive cleanup campaign throughout Honolulu, but especially within Chinatown. Most physicians in Honolulu assumed that plague, whatever its source, had probably found shelter in local refuse. Consequently, the triumvirate ordered all accumulations of garbage to be burned and all sewers to be cleaned and repaired. To signal its support of the sanitation efforts, the Honolulu Chamber of Commerce offered a modest contribution of private money to help with the cleanup. Much more was needed, however, so Emerson, Day, and Wood promptly invoked their authority to draw additional funds from the Hawaiian treasury, initially to construct a new city crematorium and a new city garbage incinerator. Before the crisis was over, the amounts drawn would soar into the millions of dollars.[33]

6

December's Debates and
"a Sad Christmas Present"

To the great relief of everyone in Honolulu, no additional plague deaths occurred in the days following the initial outbreak. The dying stopped so abruptly, in fact, that people began to doubt whether plague had really been in the city at all. Would a real epidemic of bubonic plague kill just five people in a little more than twenty-four hours, then disappear? Doubts increased when Hoffman released the result of a postmortem he performed on the body of a Hawaiian woman who expired inside Chinatown three days after the quarantine went into effect. This time he found no *pestis* bacilli and attributed the woman's death to unknown causes. Also puzzling was the behavior of a guinea pig Hoffman had injected with bacteria taken from one of the first five victims. The guinea pig continued to plod stoically around its cage, apparently unaffected by what was supposed to be a deadly dose. Though Hoffman vigorously defended his positive findings of plague in the first five victims, other European and American physicians began to question that diagnosis.[1]

"I think this [plague business] is all foolery," proclaimed the unofficial leader of these skeptical doctors in a newspaper interview. The source of that opinion, John S. McGrew, was not just another physician in town. Now seventy-four years old, he had graduated from Ohio Medical College in Cincinnati in 1847 and served as a surgeon in the Union army during the

Civil War. After the war he had taken his second wife on a world tour, but when they reached Honolulu in 1867, they decided to go no farther and settled there permanently. McGrew had been a leader among the city's Western physicians since then. In 1892 he founded the Hawaiian Medical Society, and he served as its president for the next five years.[2]

McGrew commanded a great deal of influence among Honolulu's oldest generation of American business and political elites. Passionately involved in pro-American politics, McGrew had played a role in securing the U.S.-Hawaiian reciprocity treaty of 1875, which opened the American market to Hawaiian sugar planters. He also helped the U.S. Navy obtain lease rights to Pearl Harbor in the 1880s. King Kalakaua himself called the doctor "Annexation McGrew." When the McKinley administration finally maneuvered its formal takeover of the Hawaiian Islands in 1898, the pro-American press hailed McGrew as "the Father of Annexation." Above all else, McGrew did not want the presence of plague to cast a shadow over the already contentious debate underway in Washington, D.C., about whether to grant full territorial status to Hawaii. Territorial status would consummate his political ambitions as triumphantly as the honorary vice presidency of an International Medical Congress had consummated his professional ambitions. He did not want a tiny handful of newcomers to torpedo the process—especially if they were wrong.[3]

Other less-outspoken physicians in the city joined the crusty McGrew in suggesting more discreetly that their colleagues on the Board of Health might have overreacted. Unless the presence of plague was proven beyond a doubt, the critics argued, the Board's physicians had a duty to refrain from making Hawaii look like a medically dangerous place and a responsibility to avoid crippling their city's trade by adding Honolulu to the international list of plague ports. Emerson, Day, and Wood had moved too precipitously on too little evidence, the critics argued, and they had abused their emergency powers.[4]

Old grudges and professional antipathies also surfaced. Several European physicians, who disliked the upstart Dole administration to begin with, resented the completely arbitrary delegation of absolute authority to just three doctors—all of whom were shamelessly pro-American and all of whom had gained appointment through political loyalties and personal networks. The medical outsiders saw the whole business as an abdication of civil responsibility on the part of the government and "a very dangerous experiment" undertaken with insufficient cause. Though McGrew was more likely to accuse Emerson, Day, and Wood of the opposite—being insufficiently attuned to pro-American political interests—he also resented the Board's power for personal reasons. Years earlier he had secured a government medical post for his adopted son Henri, only to have the Board publicly humiliate the family by removing Henri for incompetence.[5]

Disagreements among the city's white physicians came to a head when the Hawaiian Medical Society, which was still dominated by McGrew's allies, met in the main dining room of the prestigious Pacific Club on the evening of December 16 to discuss Honolulu's medical situation. Several doctors grumbled about the unreliability of the Board's evidence; others suggested that the cases they had seen could be explained without a diagnosis of plague. James H. Raymond spoke for several physicians when he professed no overt hostility toward bacteriology per se, but said he did not believe that standard "bacteriological methods" themselves had yet definitively proved the presence of plague—especially since Hoffman's "valiant little guinea pig" had so impolitely refused to die. The way Raymond and others like him saw the situation, Emerson, Day, and Wood were relying on nothing more than the unsubstantiated opinion of a relatively unknown young German who thought he saw through his one good eye some bacteria that looked like *pestis*.[6]

What began as a professional debate soon descended to acrimonious exchanges of personal opinion and rank speculation. Those who sided with the three doctors on the Board of Health found themselves increasingly on the defensive. At the end of the evening, the medical assembly publicly embarrassed Emerson, Day, and Wood, first by refusing to endorse Hoffman's bacteriological report on the original five plague cases, and then by voting to table a conciliatory motion that would have affirmed the temporary presence of plague at the time the quarantine was declared, even if the disease might no longer be present in the city.[7]

When the *Star* criticized the Medical Society the following day for its divisive stance and lack of support in the face of such a crucial question, Luis F. Alvarez, one of those who voted against the Board the night before, wrote a public letter to all of the city's newspapers defending his fellow skeptics. Most of the papers printed it. Unlike the other critics, Alvarez actually knew something about bacteriology, having traveled to the Johns Hopkins Medical School in 1895 to take an introductory course in the new techniques. Yet he used his experience not to defend Hoffman's findings but to suggest—with some justice—that all such examinations were necessarily judgmental, imprecise, and open to doubt. Alvarez, who also doubled as Spanish consul to the Dole government, had a large practice among Portuguese and Hawaiians employed in the sugar trade and hence a strong incentive to keep that trade vigorous. Like the editor of the

Independent, he shuddered at the possibility of headlines in the United States proclaiming "Hawaiian Sugar Tainted with Bubonic Plague," and he argued that "the Board of Health be very sure of your bacteriological tests before you insist upon a fiat that may absolutely ruin the prospects of this country just when they should be the brightest."[8]

The Medical Society meeting and the Alvarez letter revealed a division among Honolulu's white physicians that closely paralleled the division among the city's Chinese healers. On the one hand, many, but not all, of the older practitioners in both the white and the Chinese medical communities generally continued to place their faith in practical experience and personal observation, which they trusted more than microscopic examinations they did not fully understand. With no new cases breaking out, both white and Chinese traditionalists suggested that the Board of Health had erred in its diagnosis and urged Emerson, Day, and Wood to rescind their declaration of plague. The whites wanted to restore their city's healthful reputation; the Chinese wanted to liberate Chinatown.

On the other hand, many, but not all, of the younger physicians in both the white and the Chinese medical communities accepted Hoffman's bacteriological proof, and agreed with the Board of Health that the world pandemic of plague had indeed come ashore in Honolulu, at least briefly. In contrast to the traditionalists, they praised the Board for recognizing that fact and for promptly implementing the tight quarantine and aggressive cleanup campaigns that had apparently throttled the epidemic before it could do widespread damage. Tong San Kai, the physician in charge of the new Chinese hospital and Consul Yang's official medical advisor, came forward in the midst of this controversy to publicly defend the Board's actions. Like Li and Kong, Tong had been in China when plague struck there five years before, and Tong had seen the body of You Chong, the man who died at the Wing Wo Tai store. Tong was convinced that You Chong and the others had indeed died of plague. "The Health Department took hold of the situation in a manner which I feel will prevent its spreading much," opined Tong through a translator, "and it is possible they may be able to check it."[9]

Even as Honolulu's traditional physicians questioned the Board's science and sagacity, politicians and the press attacked the government's doctors for having allowed Chinatown to become so unsanitary in the first place. Even in newspapers closely allied with the Dole administration, strong editorials castigated Emerson, Day, and Wood for paying too much attention in recent years to import inspections and not nearly enough attention to enforcing the city's health and housing codes. Others placed "the final responsibility" for failing to enforce sanitary standards in Chinatown on the doorstep of "Dole and his Cabinet," since they had not provided the Board with enough resources. The Board's physicians were accused of being "too busy in the practice of their profession and the collection of fees, private and public," to pay attention to "the unsavory section" of "the city under their care." Still others accused the Board of tacitly exempting Chinatown's powerful American landlords from compliance with city hygiene requirements. Many voices blamed a faulty reporting structure for the mess in Chinatown and called for a Board of Health that would be independent of the attorney general's office. The Board even found itself embroiled in disputes over the efficacy of purported antiplague remedies being sold unscrupulously by city pharmacies to frightened citizens.[10]

Hawaiians joined the chorus of recrimination. *Ke Aloha Aina*, for example, published the observations of a man who had gained access to the quarantined zone by working as a servant in the district's cleanup operations. "The Japanese and Chinese are not the unclean ones who are spreading the plague in the city," he concluded. "Instead, it is the large land owners who rent units on a large-scale profit. These are people such as Samuel Damon, Dillingham, Keoni Kolopana and some others who sit and collect huge monthly and annual profits. The Chinese and Japanese," in the view of this Hawaiian observer, were merely "tenants trying to make a living for themselves and their children. The units [regarded as foul by the Board of Health] are convenient for the time being until they can secure more permanent residences." The Hawaiian press editorialized that large landlords should be forced to bring such units up to acceptable standards at their own expense or be compelled to pay for their destruction.[11]

After five days of anxious quarantine, medical debate, and no additional deaths, the beleaguered physicians on the Board of Health loosened their regulations. They permitted public trams to pass through Chinatown, provided they did not stop in the quarantined zone, thereby reconnecting the areas west of Nuuanu stream to the center of the city. Mail delivery resumed in Chinatown. "The danger seems to be over," speculated the city's newspapers, "and the quarantine will undoubtedly be raised within a short time." Through the Chamber of Commerce, the city's retail merchants pressed the Board to relax the quarantine as quickly as possible to leave time for last-minute Christmas shopping.[12]

Following a closed meeting on December 18, Emerson, Day, and Wood voted to terminate their week-long quarantine. Some Japanese businessmen called the Board's quick decision "careless," since they now contended—in contrast to their initial protests—that if plague bacteria had really been in the city, then they were almost certainly still lurking in the area. More pointedly, they observed that they would suffer long delays in retrieving their goods from quarantined warehouses, while their white competitors would be in a position to cash in on pent-up holiday demand just as soon as normal business resumed. Consequently, Japanese merchants again saw "racial bias" behind the Board's hasty decision to lift its emergency regulations, and they assumed that white businessmen must have bribed the Board's physicians to reopen the city on terms that favored them.[13]

The final hours of the quarantine did not pass smoothly. After rumors circulated about the mysterious death of a Chinese woman inside the quarantined district, medical inspectors broke down the door to the house where the woman's body lay and performed a postmortem examination. With palpable relief, they concluded that she had died as the result of a fall. More ominous was the case of a white teenager named Ethel Johnson, who lived on the Iwilei Road between Chinatown and the harbor. The Board physicians who examined the teenager considered her case "highly suspicious" and ordered a miniature quarantine and an armed guard placed around the Johnson house, but they did not immediately declare her a plague victim. *Ke Aloha Aina* reported that Hoffman believed Ethel did have plague, but another doctor had objected to the diagnosis "since she was a white girl, and [the other doctor] wished to save her from being grouped together with Hawaiians, Japanese and Chinese, an act which would defile the dignity of their whiteness, the people who control and rule this archipelago."[14]

If Ethel did have bubonic plague, the Board's physicians hypothesized, she probably contracted it from the human waste being hauled from the privies of Chinatown past her house to a seaside dump. As a precaution, the cleanup crews were ordered to change their routes to avoid residential areas. In any event, the girl had survived her first wave of fever, and even if she should take a turn for the worse, she lived outside the quarantined area. So the Board officially lifted the quarantine of Chinatown at noon on December 20 and permitted public activities to resume throughout the city. Newspapers likened the scene to the Oklahoma land rush as Chinatown's residents flowed back across the painted lines into the central city. Public transportation resumed its normal functions, schools reopened, and scores of ships, which had been moored for a week, cheerfully departed for Pacific destinations from Sydney to San Francisco.[15]

The citizens of Honolulu quickly resumed their normal patterns of life as newspaper headlines confidently declared, "PLAGUE STAMPED OUT." A housewife remembered that "the quarantine was raised on Chinatown and all was bustle as the merchants made up for lost time." Freighters off-loaded their cargo, schools reopened, and city merchants hoped for a last-minute Christmas rush. But Emerson, Day, and Wood, still smarting under the charges of doing too little before the plague arrived in Honolulu and too much after it showed up, remained proactive. They hoped that their prompt and decisive intervention had checked an initial onslaught of plague at home, but they remained concerned that the larger world pandemic showed no signs of abating. Plague continued to rage throughout Asia and regularly appeared in new sites from Australia to Portugal. So the three physicians realized that their city remained as vulnerable as ever. Consequently, only three hours after the quarantine officially ended, they met again with President Dole to outline additional actions designed to avoid future crises.[16]

Chief among their propositions was a massive sanitary initiative in Chinatown. Though no one made public reference to the accusations of previous dereliction leveled against the government's public health team, everyone on the Board of Health now resolved to be much more vigorous in their hygienic oversight of that district. Their plan called for an ad hoc

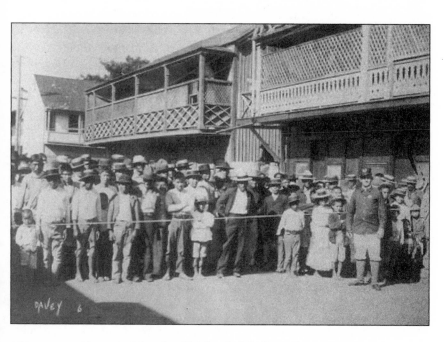

Chinatown residents awaiting the official end of the December quarantine.
Hawaii State Archives

sanitary committee to conduct a survey of what needed to be done, and they proposed a special appropriation of $100,000 to pay for it. New excavating equipment would have to be purchased, a new city incinerator would have to be constructed, two new water filtration systems would have to be installed, and new sewers and drains would have to be laid. Individual owners would be assessed the cost of bringing their private property up to sanitary standards previously set by the Board. C. B. Reynolds, who had conducted medical surveys while chief executive officer to the kingdom's Board of Health in the late 1880s and early 1890s, agreed to head the ad hoc sanitary committee for Chinatown, and he was joined by two government loyalists, Judge George R. Carter and F. B. Edwards.[17]

According to the press, most people in the city agreed in a general sense with the Board of Health's basic premise: improving the sanitary condition of Chinatown should be a civic priority. How could they disagree? But serious questions surfaced immediately. No one knew for certain whether the Board of Health could still draw at will upon the treasury after the plague emergency ended, or how the continued depletion of the republic's treasury might impact the territorial debates in Washington. Both wealthy landlords and marginal business owners inside Chinatown were leery of a sudden and rather arbitrary policy that was being promulgated by a nonelective board and might cost them large sums of money to improve property they already considered hygienically adequate. Political opponents of the Dole government feared the proposal as a raid upon the treasury and a way of steering lucrative government contracts toward friends of the Dole administration. Chinese consul Yang, who had supported the Board during the quarantine, now announced his formal opposition to the peremptory sanitation plan.[18]

Even as the press debated how to pay for the cleaning of Chinatown, Emerson, Day, and Wood began to receive alarming reports of more deaths. On December 23, they learned that Ethel Johnson had succumbed at her home. The next day a twenty-seven-year-old Chinese laborer known as Ah Fong, who had lived in Chinatown during the quarantine, was found dead in the adjoining Palama district. Autopsies confirmed what Emerson, Day, and Wood feared most: both victims had certainly died of plague. They also learned that some traditional Chinese healers had apparently resumed the practice of covering up plague deaths to avoid mandatory cremation, which raised the possibility of even more new cases than the ones they knew about. Though sorely tempted to take punitive action against the Chinese practitioners implicated in the mortuary cover-ups, the doctors decided not to provoke open confrontation and backed off. Besides, the next day was Christmas; perhaps things would improve.[19]

December's Debates and "a Sad Christmas Present"

Emerson and his wife Sarah were sitting at their dining room table the following afternoon when a knock at the front door interrupted their Christmas dinner. The same thing happened at Day's house and at Wood's. A twenty-four-year-old Chinese laborer named Chong Mon Dow had been found dead in Chinatown, and the people who found him had sent messengers to the homes of the Board's three physicians. All three doctors rushed off to inspect the body. Another impromptu autopsy confirmed what they already knew: his lymph system was bursting with *pestis*.

The three physicians returned to their downtown office and reluctantly faced the fact that the epidemic had indeed returned. Christmas or not, they now felt they had no choice but to declare Honolulu again under attack from bubonic plague—which they solemnly did that afternoon in a formal vote. To do otherwise, they resolved, would be cowardly and dangerous, since none of them—and none of the physicians working with them—could any longer seriously doubt "that these cases with hemorrhagic buboes are cases of plague." Even some of the physicians who had publicly questioned the Board's diagnoses during the first wave of cases now reluctantly conceded that Hoffman's earlier bacteriological conclusions must have been accurate.[20]

The Dole administration immediately summoned all foreign consuls in the city to the capitol building and officially informed them that Honolulu was once again an "infected port" under international protocols. Carmichael dispatched similar notification by ship to his counterparts at the Marine Hospital Service in San Francisco; they would have to guard that port of entry to the United States and decide whether or not to continue to send American troops to the Philippines by way of Hawaii. As spokesman for the interim government of an American possession, Dole's consul-general also felt obliged to send formal notification to the U.S. State Department in Washington. Everyone realized that this was "a very serious matter and a very sad Christmas present for Hawaii."[21]

By official decree, the "existing government" reaffirmed the absolute emergency powers of the medical triumvirate throughout the Hawaiian archipelago, effective December 26, 1899. Sheriffs on the outer islands were formally declared agents of the Honolulu Board of Health. The decree reasserted the physicians' power to quarantine individual properties on an ad hoc basis and larger districts as they saw fit. Fearing that a general quarantine of Chinatown might be reinstated at any moment, Japanese and Chinese were reported to be "excitedly running with sachels [*sic*] to the homes of family members outside the [Chinatown district]." They were worried "that their homes will [again] come under quarantine and that they will lose their jobs."[22]

For the next several days, Emerson, Day, and Wood wrestled with the problems already at hand, considered various steps they might take, met with many groups to hear different points of view, and tried to grope their way toward a coherent set of public policies. The first problem they addressed was the alleged concealment of plague victims among the Chinese. They sent word to "the merchants and leading men of the Chinese colony" that they needed "assistance in suppressing the plague" and arranged for a meeting on the afternoon of December 26. With Wood's friend W. H. Crawford acting as interpreter, the Board's physicians assured the Chinese representatives that they were not being singled out— cremations were being performed solely on the basis of public safety. They reminded the Chinese that "only last Saturday [when] a white girl [Ethel Johnson] died of the plague, we cremated her just the same as we did in the cases of your countrymen." They also squelched a rumor circulating in the sharply factionalized Chinese community that Consul Yang was complicit in the decision to cremate earlier Chinese victims because they had not been among his political supporters.[23]

By the end of the meeting, a rough agreement had emerged. Chinese physicians could continue to treat all sicknesses in their community, with the exception of plague. Plague patients would be removed to a special plague hospital set up by the Board of Health. The bodies of plague victims would be given to the Board of Health for disposal, but Consul Yang would be formally notified prior to cremation, in order to verify the identity of the deceased. To partly offset the horror of cremation, Emerson, Day, and Wood promised to return the bones and ashes of plague victims to the families or friends of the deceased. In another shrewd concession, the physicians won key support from the Chinese business community by agreeing to fumigate any of their suspect merchandise at public expense if the businessmen, in turn, provided the warehouse space for that process to take place. Chinese merchants had lost thousands of dollars during the mid-December quarantine and had come to the meeting fearful of more costly embargoes in the future.[24]

Hoping that the special meeting had assuaged the city's principal Chinese leaders, the three physicians turned to other issues. As the first step in their proposed sanitizing of the Chinatown district, they ordered an immediate reinspection to determine the feasibility of a new sewage system. Since several of the physicians working with Emerson, Day, and Wood shared their long-standing suspicion that rats were somehow involved in the spread of plague—even though none of them knew exactly how—the triumvirate announced a bounty of ten cents apiece on dead rats.

The Board also issued a circular printed in English, Hawaiian, Portuguese, Japanese, and Chinese, outlining "Precautions Against Bubonic Plague." The circular began by asserting the common wisdom that "Plague germs flourish in filth, in garbage and in damp, dark or foul places." Consequently, cleanliness was essential. Cuts and scratches should be covered; food should be well cooked. The circular also invoked Kitasato's soil theories: "Dr. Kitasato, the celebrated plague specialist," stated the circular, believes that plague frequently attacks people from the ground up. "Therefore," warned the Board's physicians, "it is dangerous to go barefoot in times like this; wear shoes." Finally, admonished the circular, "destroy all the rats and vermin on your premises and the danger of plague will become less."[25]

Barely a day and a half into the post-Christmas emergency, the situation inside Chinatown seemed to be deteriorating rapidly, particularly among the Chinese. After angry protestors threatened Li Khai Fai for his continuing cooperation with the Board of Health, the triumvirate felt the need to post permanent police protection outside Li's Chinatown home. Handbills urging independent resistance against white medical policies and against Consul Yang's cremation concessions were tacked up around Chinatown. Nervous white businessmen urged Emerson, Day, and Wood to crack down on "the agitators who are inciting the Chinese." They favored the use of live ammunition if necessary.[26]

Some Chinese continued to conceal suspected cases of plague not only from white medical inspectors but also from neighbors who complied with the consul's agreement. Other Chinese had begun to expel ailing countrymen from their midst, fearing that plague cases might provoke ad hoc quarantines around the houses and stores where they lived and worked. As a result, the dead bodies of Chinese workers were discovered around the city in apparently random public places. In one sad case, a body was found lying outside the locked gates of the Chinese hospital.[27]

Vice-Consul Gu still remembered that last incident many years later. A Chinese doctor had decided he could do no more for a patient named Chen, so he advised the man's friends to tell him to go to the Wai Wah Yee Yuen hospital in the Palama district and hope for the best. Though the doctor dared not tell Chen's friends, he feared that Chen might infect the entire hospital if he lived long enough to be admitted. So the doctor first sent secret word to hospital director Tong strongly advising against the admission of Chen, then notified Board headquarters that he had heard rumors about a possible plague case in the neighborhood of the hospital. To verify the rumor, Board physicians went to Wai Wah Yee Yuen, where they found

Chen's lifeless body huddled against the hospital fence. His remains were removed for immediate cremation. Emerson, Day, and Wood regarded incidents like that—however understandable given the constraints facing their Chinese colleagues—as dangerously irresponsible, since they involved the dispersal of patients full of *pestis*.[28]

To make matter worse, discouraged health inspectors found several sites inside Chinatown that seemed more unsanitary than they had initially appeared during the emergency survey just a week earlier. Indeed, preliminary reports from the ad hoc sanitary committee suggested that the Board's grand plans for vigorous sanitary improvements and sewer construction in the Chinatown district would likely be more difficult to implement and more costly to finance than initially imagined. The cleanup could probably not be accomplished quickly, or at least not quickly enough to quash the burgeoning crisis at hand.

Among the few bright spots from the Board's point of view was the active cooperation of Honolulu's most influential Japanese physicians. Under the Westernizing mandates of the Meiji government back home, these doctors had been trained to approach medical issues in much the same way their American counterparts approached them. They revered Kitasato as a national hero. Mitamura Toshiyuki, who had been practicing in the Hawaiian Islands since 1888 and had strong ties to many American physicians through their mutual commitment to the Christian social movement, coordinated the flow of medical information from the Japanese community to the Board of Health. He and five Japanese colleagues organized a team of thirty-one community inspectors to conduct rigorous patrols throughout the Japanese portions of Chinatown. Far from concealing suspicious cases, much less suspicious deaths, the Japanese physicians systematically referred all patients with the slightest hint of plague symptoms to the Board's plague hospital at Kakaako. Mitamura also visited the hospital every day to help care for the Japanese-speaking patients. When many of those patients proved not to have plague, they were released to their homes and to their regular physicians for further treatment.[29]

Through the afternoon of December 27, the Board physicians were "kept busy" with an abrupt surge of new cases, mostly in Chinatown. By the end of the day, they were convinced of the need for quick and decisive action. Shortly after midnight, in the early hours of December 28, they formally re-mobilized the Hawaiian national guard and formally reinstated a complete quarantine of the Chinatown district. This time the triumvirate vowed a regimen "far more strict than the last quarantine" and ordered the national guard to patrol the periphery of the quarantined zone with bayonets fixed. By 3:00 A.M. the cordon was in place.[30]

The midnight quarantine drew angry protests and ugly threats the next morning. The English-language press suspected a young Chinese lawyer of actively organizing protests among his countrymen both inside and outside Chinatown, though the press did not know for sure who the young radical was. Three different groups of Japanese men disregarded the admonitions of the Japanese consul and attempted "to run the guard," only to be captured by mounted police and returned to the quarantine district. The staff of *Ke Aloha Aina* sympathized with their Hawaiian friends caught inside the zone. "While people . . . were sleeping in their homes, they suddenly became surrounded by government troops who were sent to guard the area with their rifles projecting everywhere. Residents were panic-stricken, but helpless to defend themselves from the will of the government." Like the Board of Health itself, *Ke Aloha Aina* blamed the reimposed quarantine at least in part upon the Chinese practice of sending plague victims out of Chinatown to die elsewhere.[31]

Following initial resistance, order was restored inside the quarantined zone over the course of the day. The United Chinese Society organized a committee of twelve under the direction of Lin Shen Chow to emulate the voluntary inspections being undertaken by the Japanese. The society doubtless hoped that such actions might forestall the reimposition of outside inspectors, whose activities had caused so much tension during the earlier quarantine. Learning from recent experience, the triumvirate immediately ordered the delivery of fresh meat, fresh produce, and poi to residents inside the quarantined zone, at government expense.[32]

Emerson, Day, and Wood were convinced they had acted none too soon. Even as guards were being posted, they apprehended a gravely ill Chinese laborer attempting to slip out of the quarantined zone. He was forcibly removed to the plague hospital at Kakaako, where he quickly succumbed. An autopsy, performed by Kobayashi Sanzaburo and Mori Iga, the two principal directors of Honolulu's Japanese hospital, confirmed bubonic plague as the cause of death. On the same day, Hoffman's slides also confirmed the death of a young Hawaiian boy named Maunakina as plague. Skeptics could grumble all they wanted, businessmen could wish things were otherwise, politicians could worry about Hawaii's image, and the residents of Chinatown could protest their quarantine; but the three physicians on the Board of Health were now fully convinced they had the world epidemic of bubonic plague on their hands—and the brief quarantine in the middle of December had not snuffed it out.[33]

7

The Decision to Use Fire

The grim "Christmas present" of 1899 put tremendous pressure on Emerson, Day, and Wood. With the reconfirmation of their absolute emergency powers came an expectation that they would not only stop the epidemic from decimating the city in the short run, but also extinguish the plague so completely that it would be unable to establish a permanent Hawaiian presence. Exactly how to achieve either of those goals, however, was far from obvious. Every day that passed brought additional deaths, and people throughout the city were beginning to realize that they were all trapped together in the middle of the ocean with no place to run.

By reinstating the Chinatown quarantine, the three physicians hoped to confine the disease to a manageable area, as they thought they had done two weeks earlier. But confinement without some program of eradication was pointless, even dangerous, since everyone confined inside the zone with the *pestis* bacteria remained at risk. So Emerson, Day, and Wood turned to the ad hoc sanitary committee they had appointed before the plague reappeared, hoping those men had some ideas about eliminating the conditions that *pestis* seemed to require.

On the afternoon of December 29, the three members of the ad hoc committee met with the three physicians at the Board of Health office. Emerson, Day, and Wood were encouraged to learn that the committee members had already developed a detailed list of ten proposals for sanitizing the Chinatown slum. The proposals ranged from "the immediate building of a garbage crematory," through extensive site grading and sewage treatment, to revised zoning laws with sharp teeth. The committee recognized that many of their proposals were potentially expensive for both Chinatown property owners and the public treasury, but they assured the physicians that they had given their assignment a great deal of thought and tried to consider both the present crisis and Honolulu's future. "With our large ocean trade we shall always be exposed to contagion," they argued, so in the long run the city would be ahead to spend whatever it took to make sure Chinatown was "in a condition to repel disease, and to prevent [diseases from] securing a foothold rather than undergo the loss caused by quarantine regulations, the interruption of trade, and the prevention of the free flow of commodities, which is essential to the life of commerce as well as the very existence of [our] community."[1]

Fully persuaded—and glad to have a coherent plan of action—Emerson, Day, and Wood approved the ad hoc committee's proposals and began to allot funds to implement them. The amounts they authorized were substantial, far in excess of their initial estimate of $100,000. Even though the earlier figure had triggered taxpayer protests and editorial debates, the three physicians now unflinchingly approved "$120,000 for water filtration plants, $25,000 for a garbage crematory, $80,000 for opening new streets and alleys, and $300,000 for extending the sewer system." In a single afternoon, the "mission boy" public health officer and the two medical partners from Ohio launched the most massive public works projects in Hawaiian history. The sums they drew from the republic's treasury in half an hour would never have been authorized by the civilian legislature under normal circumstances. But these were hardly normal circumstances. Indeed, the three physicians wondered whether the sanitation program by itself—even on this unprecedented scale—was enough. Was there anything else they could, or should, consider?[2]

To address that question, Emerson, Day, and Wood called a special session of the Board of Health for the following evening, December 30. Around the table with them sat titular Board president Henry Cooper, the republic's attorney general who seldom attended the Board's regular meetings, and George W. Smith, a civilian member of the Board. C. B. Reynolds, who had overseen preparation of the sanitary proposals accepted the day before, attended as an invited guest. Cooper called the group to order at 7 P.M., and introduced another invited guest, Lorrin Thurston, the man who had masterminded the Hawaiian annexation movement and who still served as the republic's principal political strategist.

Everyone around the table knew Thurston well and had worked with him in many capacities before; and the broad-gauged Thurston, in turn, had plenty of prior experience in matters of medical policy and public health. Emerson remembered serving with Thurston on the old Board of Health under Kalakaua; Day had been part of Thurston's inner circle since Day's admission to the secret Annexationist Club that toppled Liliuokalani; Wood knew Thurston not only as a close personal friend but also as the mastermind of Hawaii's American takeover. No doubt concerned about what the on-again-off-again plague reports from Honolulu might be doing to Hawaii's chances for full territorial status, Thurston had decided to get involved. In the words of the *Friend*, a paper that greatly admired him and agreed with his agenda for the future of Hawaii, Thurston wanted to put his "great organizing and directing ability" at the disposal of his friends on the Board and to offer some suggestions for "efficient dealing with the enemy."[3]

Thurston began by summarizing the fears and criticisms then circulating among the dominant Americans in Honolulu. Most of the latter seemed afraid that the Board was acting too deliberately and too cautiously in the face of a grave threat, not only to the immediate health of the population but also to the long-term future of Hawaiian development. Everyone knew that the pandemic had been lingering in Hong Kong for five years. Should the same thing happen in Honolulu, the result would be nothing less than "a ruinous catastrophe." Everything the annexationists had worked for would be put at risk if bubonic plague were allowed to become endemic. The maritime economy of the archipelago might be crippled for years. Consequently, Thurston had come to urge "stronger measures" than any taken so far.[4]

Thurston had recently read in the journal *Nineteenth Century* an analysis of the way the current plague epidemic was affecting a city in Portugal. The essay confirmed his view that conventional quarantines by themselves had done little to quell the disease elsewhere; in fact, they probably increased the likelihood of additional cases among the already vulnerable people confined to infected areas. Logically then, Thurston believed, the Honolulu Board should not confine people inside plague zones, but should remove them and quarantine them elsewhere long enough to know they were not plague carriers themselves, while trying to destroy—by whatever means necessary—the sources of plague left behind.[5]

During informal discussions with Wood prior to the Board's formal session, Thurston and the doctor had both agreed that fire was the one and only sure method of eradicating the otherwise apparently tenacious plague bacilli. Drawing the obvious conclusion, Thurston now suggested to his longtime associates around the table that they begin removing people from known plague sites for their own good, placing the evacuees in safe quarantine zones, and then burning the vacated sites, along with any contents that might harbor bacteria, in order to destroy the *pestis* known to be lurking there. Thurston left in abeyance the difficult question of trying to define the appropriate dimensions of a plague site: a room, a single building, the surrounding block, a whole neighborhood, or perhaps an entire district?[6]

To advance the discussion, Cooper offered a test case. Along with two physicians and two city surveyors, he had inspected a set of interconnected buildings where a Chinese man known simply as Ahi had died of plague. The entire inspection party had concluded that most of the buildings at the site were incapable of being effectively cleaned or disinfected in the manner authorized the previous day. Nor could fresh water or sewers be run to them. Since there was every reason to believe that "the whole block is infected around Ahi's place," Cooper proposed relocating the other residents of that block to a special quarantine camp elsewhere in the city and burning all but four or five salvageable structures. Cooper recognized the gravity of his proposal. Even "to discuss this matter," he observed, raised a "question of policy."

When civilian George Smith expressed qualms about the legality of Cooper's proposal, the attorney general countered with a remarkably frank statement. According to the minutes of the meeting, he claimed that there were "two ways of going about [the task of sanitizing the block in question]. The legal one was to serve notice on the owners and occupants for abatement of nuisances[,] giving them time to [make improvements]; the other way was to go in and destroy the unsanitary structures[,] leaving the matter of damages to be settled later." Cooper strongly advocated the more draconian course of action. "The Board had been charged with being negligent for not adopting drastic measures. These criticisms may be misunderstood abroad and cause far reaching consequences endangering the commerce of the country." With the stakes so high, the government's chief legal officer was announcing to the Board that he had no intention of abiding by legal technicalities. Extraordinary crises justified extraordinary actions.[7]

A defender of traditional property rights, Smith again demurred. "Follow the course of the law and give [property owners] notice," he urged his colleagues on the Board. "I think it is ridiculous," he asserted, "to burn all these people out. Condemn these buildings according to law." Smith was confident that ordinary condemnation proceedings would force property owners, some of whom were his friends, to make necessary improvements. He was also concerned about how the Board was going to provide for a potentially large number of displaced persons with little or no lead time to prepare either temporary or permanent housing arrangements.[8]

The three physicians felt frustrated by a lack of alternative approaches. Bacteriological laboratories around the world were continuing to work on various antiplague serums, but none had yet produced anything of proven frontline value in the struggle against the *pestis* bacterium. A number of prophylactic preparations were in production, but their effectiveness was hotly debated, not only by those who had tested them in the field but also by rival producers and nonbelievers. British experiments in India with the best known of those prophylactic preparations, the so-called Haffkine's serum, had been inconclusive. Kitasato himself claimed no more than a 50-percent success rate with a preventive serum he had developed and tried in Japan. Moreover, no one in the world was claiming to have found a therapeutic antidote to give people who already had the disease. And even if promising products were about to appear somewhere in the world, they could not possibly reach Honolulu by ship for another four to six weeks. Death tolls could soar in that length of time, and the disease might become so thoroughly entrenched that outside help would be of little value.[9]

The Board's physicians were further handicapped in December 1899 by the fact that none of the world's bacteriologists, and certainly no one in Honolulu, really knew much about the behavior of the *pestis* bacteria they had identified five years earlier. They had an exact portrait of what the enemy looked like, so they knew when it was present; but they still had remarkably little information about the enemy's essential qualities, much less how it was getting from person to person. How long could the bacteria survive in food, or in merchandise, or in water? How much heat and cold could the bacteria tolerate? Were other animals besides rats susceptible to plague? Could the bacteria live in the ground, and if so, for how long? The answers to such questions were just not available to the doctors sitting around the table that late December evening, or to their colleagues elsewhere in the world.[10]

As with the case of serums, Emerson, Day, and Wood knew that earlier efforts to kill plague bacteria in noninvasive ways, including some they had tried themselves, had gone quite badly. They were also familiar with British efforts in India to deploy a host of different gaseous disinfectants and acid washes against *pestis*. In addition to being quite costly, those materials had proved awkwardly inefficient to apply. But worst of all, according to reports in the international public health journals, money and manpower aside, none of them had proved capable of thoroughly eradicating ambient bacilli under real-life conditions. Thus in the opinion of most experts, including the authoritative Kitasato, the sole weapon absolutely certain to destroy *pestis* was fire, which is why the Board had ordered the cremation of plague victims from the outset and why Thurston and Cooper, with Wood's tacit support, were now proposing the use of fire in Honolulu.[11]

Given the seriousness of the situation and the lack of alternatives, Emerson declared himself ready to accept the new policy implied in Cooper's proposal. The veteran public health officer had trusted Thurston's judgment at the time of the kahuna crisis, and he was prepared to trust him again. "I am willing to go right ahead and take all the responsibility and burn anything and do anything that is necessary," opined the senior physician at the table. "I think that is the proper policy of the Board." Day quickly concurred. To stop the epidemic, he said, the three of them had a responsibility "to remove the people from the infected houses," even if that meant destroying "many of the houses in Chinatown."

Wood, who had already conferred with Thurston unofficially, put his support into the form of a motion. Henceforth, "all wooden buildings in which a case of plague occurs, and all wooden buildings in immediate communication therewith" would be "burned as soon as possible, precautions being taken to prevent the fire spreading," and people living in such buildings would "be immediately removed . . . to quarantine quarters." Special provisions were made for brick and stone buildings, which might be saved and disinfected in other ways; for various sorts of furnishings inside condemned buildings, depending upon whether or not the physicians thought they were likely to harbor bacteria; for the disposal of personal items, some of which could be fumigated and returned to their owners; for damage appraisals, which would be necessary at some future point when residents would be compensated for their losses; and for many other matters, including recompense for personal items like family photographs and treasured heirlooms that might have to be incinerated lest they harbor bacteria.[12]

With all of the others determined to adopt the new policy, Smith acquiesced. Signaling support, he moved that the block inspected by Cooper's team be declared "an infected district and a source of filth and a cause of sickness; and that all dwellings, building, stores, structures or other enclosures situated thereon, be destroyed by fire; saving and excepting such buildings as may be reserved therefrom which are shown on a map of such district by red lines." The voting members of the Board unanimously adopted Smith's motion, the first of what would become many similar condemnations. The order could not be executed until assessors had gone through the block and alternative housing had been found. Nonetheless, invoking their emergency powers, the Honolulu Board of Health had decided to begin the twentieth century by removing residents from their homes and incarcerating them in quarantine camps and by burning private property in defense of the public's health.[13]

For the record, Wood made clear that the Board itself would control all aspects of the new policy and maintain direct oversight of all relocation camps. Emerson urged his colleagues to begin requisitioning various public sites and official buildings for use "as quarantine quarters for people from infected houses." Probably in direct response to editorials in the press that accused the quarantine of rapidly descending to the level of "opera bouffe," Day moved to strengthen the city's guard stations and maintain public order. The group dispersed at 9:45 P.M., having agreed in less than three hours on a dramatic escalation in their war against bubonic plague. Day broke the tension by remarking to his colleagues that "the community would have said the Board 'had gone crazy'" if they had adopted these policies six months earlier.[14]

The decision to burn plague sites was a bold departure, since the deliberate use of fire against plague was not—contrary to intuitive assumptions—a common practice prior to the global pandemic of the 1890s. To be sure, goods and clothes were sometimes burned in earlier plague epidemics, since many people feared such items might somehow convey disease. Islamic medicine had used smoke from specific types of aromatic wood in hopes of warding off plagues. Unintended fires appear in retrospect to have inadvertently helped suppress plagues, as happened famously in London in 1666. And without a doubt, the occasional building was sometimes intentionally torched, though usually for symbolic reasons, or for scapegoating purposes, not as part of a systematic public health policy. But for the most part, buildings were valuable assets, not to be destroyed cavalierly, especially when there was no reason to believe that destroying them would affect the spread of the disease.

Only with the current pandemic—and the bacteriological understanding of disease—did public health officials try the tactic of deliberately and systematically burning plague sites. Bacteriological experts believed that *pestis* could lurk inside buildings, beneath floorboards, and behind walls, so burning would incinerate any bacteria still hiding there. The precedent best known to members of the Honolulu Board of Health was the British use of fire to disinfect a small portion of the Taipingshan district of Hong Kong in 1894. Even there, the British had targeted just 6.25 acres and 384 houses, a fifth of which had experienced at least three plague deaths apiece. Moreover, the British had first demolished the buildings, then burned the rubble.[15]

In 1899, surprisingly few buildings in Honolulu were regarded as genuine assets. As the Board's physicians explicitly recognized and openly discussed, rising urban land values meant that most lots in the city would be worth more without their existing structures than with them. This was especially true inside the Chinatown district, where a high percentage of poorly constructed buildings occupied potentially prime commercial land immediately adjacent to the harbor. Emerson, Day, and Wood never consciously acted on such economic premises. Quite the contrary—they were bitterly annoyed that any burnings they undertook might paradoxically reward owners who had flaunted the city's building and hygienic codes, by increasing the value of their land at public expense. Nonetheless, selective burning, even on a rather large scale if necessary, seemed economically less destructive in burgeoning Honolulu on the eve of the twentieth century than it had seemed in most other cities in the past.[16]

To the Honolulu physicians' credit, they also stepped up their search for less destructive ways to rid buildings of bacteria. They continued to experiment with various forms of fumigation (usually with burning sulfur), with disinfecting compounds (especially formalin), and with various acid washes (testing different concentrations of each). But their ongoing efforts and experiments continued to yield either inconclusive or downright discouraging results. So, in their view, fire remained their only completely reliable option. The U.S. Army doctor assigned to Camp McKinley just outside Honolulu had already reached the same conclusion independently. "In my opinion," wrote Blair D. Taylor to his superiors in Washington near the end of December, "Chinatown will have to be burned up and rebuilt on a sanitary basis before the plague can be stamped out. Such a course, I understand, is now being contemplated by the authorities."[17]

The three physicians made the first public demonstration of their new policy on Sunday morning, December 31, 1899. At 11:00 A.M. they met three local businessmen who had agreed to constitute an ad hoc "Board of Appraisers." Together the six crossed into the quarantined zone and headed for an adjoining pair of two-story buildings, where Day had previously discovered a Chinese man named Ah Kau dead from plague. Emerson, Day, and Wood inspected the buildings, formally condemned them as a plague site unable to be disinfected in any ordinary fashion, and declared that they would have to be incinerated.[18]

After the buildings were evacuated, the appraisers made their estimates, and an order was sent to the nearby Chinatown fire station. At 3:00 P.M. firemen ignited the complex, which quickly burned to the ground. Some 85 occupants of the complex, "Chinese, Japanese, and Hawaiians," according to the Board's official record, "were taken to a new Quarantine station at Kakaako, where they will be supplied and fed." Monday morning papers carried extensive coverage of the event, thus confirming rumors that had circulated through the New Year's weekend. Lest there be any doubt, the Board ordered additional burnings each of the next two days in the block where another Chinese man, Quon Wo Quon, had died of plague on New Year's Eve. Less than a month earlier, the "existing government" in Honolulu had been happily preparing to welcome the twentieth century with altogether different fireworks.[19]

The English-language press immediately and enthusiastically endorsed the Board's decision to begin targeted burning. The pro-trade *Commercial Advertiser* heartily approved the concept of "fighting the devil with fire" and believed that "destruction is the only certain disinfection." "Expensive this will be," conceded that paper, "but the cost to Hawaii in dollars and cents alone, if the plague is not stamped out within the next thirty days, will

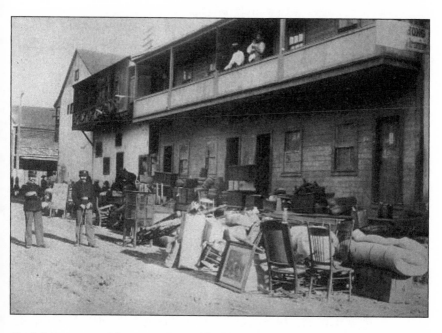

Goods being removed from a condemned building. Hawaii State Archives

pay for two Chinatowns and the Hawaiian national debt thrown in." The *Friend*, a paper that summarized events for the missionary community, was glad to see that the Board had decided to burn "the filthy tenements where the disease has appeared." According to the *Friend*, public health alone, even if plague was not upon the city's doorstep, justified the destruction of such inhumane and unsanitary situations. The greedy owners of such properties had shown no sensitivity to the patently obvious need for hygienic improvements.[20]

The *Hawaiian Gazette*, though no particular ally of the government, believed fervently that the fire policy was essential to the city's salvation and praised the combined pressure of Honolulu's newspapers for bestirring the Board into actions that finally seemed commensurate with an onslaught of the dreaded bubonic plague. "The cost of burning down whole blocks of houses, if necessary, for the public good and to save life will not be objected to by thoughtful people," argued *Austin's Hawaiian Weekly*, "even if it increases taxation." The *Evening Bulletin* heartily agreed, urging complete support for the new policy, warning people not to get carried away by rumors, and dismissing with contempt "the suggestion by a contemporary that consideration of politics influenced the Board." Perhaps most surprising of all was a lead editorial in the anti-Dole *Independent*. Two days after the first fire, that paper commended none other than Lorrin Thurston himself for spurring "our very lame Board of Health" into proper and forceful action. Two days after that, the editor followed up by assuring the Dole administration that it "need not fear attack from any party even if they spend every cent in the treasury to again render our city pure and healthy."[21]

Although the English-language press was overwhelmingly in favor of the new fire policy, Chinatown property owners themselves expressed grave reservations that quickly turned into legal protests. While removing old buildings might increase land values in the long run, they reasoned, the process would be economically disastrous in the short run. They would have no income for a minimum of several months; they would have to replace inventory and equipment at higher prices; and unless they were willing to sell the land, they would have to pony up a great deal of additional capital if they wanted to replace their lost buildings with better structures.

A large portion of the property inside Chinatown was owned by wealthy white investors from outside the district, who leased their properties to the residents. Those owners included the Hawaii Land Company, the Silvera Estate, and a number of white absentee landlords and investment trusts based in San Francisco. The Bishop Estate, a powerful corporate entity that controlled huge concentrations of land and capital throughout Hawaii, also owned substantial amounts of property in Chinatown. Most of the individuals involved in these real estate corporations would normally be counted among the Dole government's strongest supporters, but the "existing government's" Board of Health seemed now to be turning on them. Lawyers for those corporate owners quickly joined the district's individual owners, some of whom were Chinese and Japanese, in protests against what they considered the Board's arbitrary actions. In some cases the outside owners also enlisted the support of their Chinatown lessees, who would lose their places of business if the owners lost their buildings.[22]

In formal letters to the Board, Chinatown property owners challenged the suspension of ordinary legal processes. Enoch Johnson, one of the white owners, expressed the basic contention of many others: "I do hereby protest against the action of the Board of Health as it is contrary to the Constitution." The law firm that represented the Hawaii Land Company agreed. The Board's proposed actions, in their view, were "contrary to the law and Constitution, especially Article 12 of the Constitution of the Republic of Hawaii, which is the same as the Constitution of the United

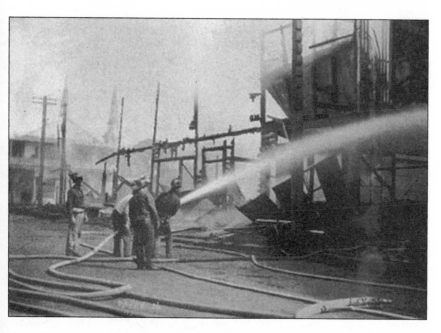

At the scene of a controlled burn in early January. Hawaii State Archives

States of America." Others went beyond expression of legal qualms to threaten members of the Board as individuals. One irate owner, for example, vowed to hold "each and every person [on the Board of Health] . . . personally liable for damages." Attorneys for several other owners likewise prepared to sue the three physicians separately "for the loss and damage" suffered by their clients and to indict the doctors for "flagrant violation . . . and prostitution of powers."[23]

Reactions from within the quarantined district itself varied widely. Most Japanese physicians continued to comply with the Board's edicts by sending anyone suspected of having plague symptoms to the plague hospital for observation. But many Japanese residents in Chinatown stopped cooperating with their own physicians, since referral might now result in the relocation of family members to a quarantine camp and the destruction of their hard-earned property. After a week of sending patients to Kakaako, Mitamura had to be "saved from serious assault at the hands of 35 Japanese" by other Japanese in the neighborhood. In just "a matter of seconds," over two hundred residents appeared at the scene of the altercation, clear evidence of the high tensions inside Chinatown. Ominously, the attack had been organized by three men who had served as inspectors during the first quarantine, but who now saw cooperation with the Board of Health as a threat to Japanese property. The instigators were later arrested and incarcerated in one of the city's detention camps. In another incident, the Japanese residents of a rooming house being inspected for possible condemnation threw a trunk at one of the Board-appointed doctors at the site, injuring his arm. Many Japanese property owners signed protest petitions alleging both discrimination on the part of the white Board and the illegality of such arbitrary actions against both people and property.[24]

In an effort to maintain order and work with the Board as much as possible under the circumstances, Japanese consul Saito Miki coordinated a central system for recording potential Japanese damage claims. Prominent Japanese who lived outside the quarantine district gathered themselves together, initially as the Japanese Society, in order to help compensate "fellow-countrymen in consequence of [losses incurred in] the sanitary fires." Out of these cooperative efforts developed some of Hawaii's most enduring Japanese charitable organizations.[25]

At least according to the English-language press, most Hawaiians inside the quarantined district appeared to be cooperating with the Board's policies, though protests over food supplies continued. One Hawaiian who had a family of six children told the press that they received four pounds of poi and half a pound of meat per day. "He says he is not to be blamed for the plague, nor is his family, and he is very desirous to learn how a member of the Board of Health would feel if placed under such circumstances on such a diet." Like others displaced by the burning of their residences, Hawaiians resented the implication that they were somehow at fault. When a site was condemned, "men were taken as if prisoners of war by lines of military guards and women were taken away by wagon under guard to be placed under quarantine."[26]

Hawaiians also protested the transporting of people to resettlement camps in the same wagons that were used to carry sick patients to the special hospital and dead plague victims to the crematorium. Their actions forced an end to that practice. The dowager queen allowed her estate to be converted to a resettlement camp for any Hawaiians forced to relocate, and Hawaiian cooperation was also enhanced by the Board's ongoing efforts to explain its policies in the Hawaiian language and by the use of Hawaiian police to deal with Hawaiians under quarantine. Hawaiians remained alert, however, to their material losses and prepared to sue for their property and leaseholder rights. They did not want to be left "like victims of the 'a'o [shearwater] bird, standing naked on the cliffside" and at the mercy of "government leaders blinded by money."[27]

The most vigorous opposition to the Board's fire policies from inside Chinatown flared up from the Chinese community. A fresh round of posters appeared, threatening death to agents of the Board and to Chinese doctors who continued to work with them. In defense of Chinese property, Consul Yang even agreed to cooperate with his reform-minded opponents in the United Chinese Society. On the day after the first fire, Yang arrived at the Board's office to present a list of demands: twenty-four-hour notice prior to any burning, assurance of suitable quarters for all those who might be displaced, and full compensation for all property losses. The three physicians acceded to the first two points and promised negotiations, once the crisis was over, regarding the third.[28]

Many Chinese property owners also organized protests of their own and, like their white and corporate counterparts, quickly retained lawyers to represent them before any courts or governmental agencies that might be willing to listen. Several wrote individually to the Board, each denying that his particular property was a health threat and asking that his goods be spared from the general policy. The Chinese consulate and the United Chinese Society also prepared and distributed broadsides urging business owners to keep carefully itemized lists of their property so that they could file claims for compensation later.[29]

The United Chinese Society also prepared formal preprinted petitions against the burning of any Chinese property and circulated them throughout the Chinese sections of Chinatown. The petition signed by ten Chinese property holders in block 2 was typical: "We recognize the serious condition of affairs at the present time and pledge ourselves to do everything possible to assist the Board of Health in stamping out the plague," avowed the petitioners. "We are ready to remodel, disinfect and fumigate, or do anything that the Board may direct toward the cleaning of any premises in this block." The petition then urged that the fire policy not be enforced on that block. The residents of seven other blocks, 155 individuals altogether, submitted identical, preprinted petitions, with the same avowals and the same requests for exemption. Among the signers were Yim Quon, president of the United Chinese Society, and Wa Ha Pau, editor of the *Chinese Chronicle*.[30]

When the Board of Health first implemented the fire policy, the "existing government" made no public statement about it. But in the face of mounting protests and the threat of personal lawsuits, Smith and the three physicians asked to meet with Dole and his top advisors. In their own words, the Board members "wanted the support of the Cabinet and the people in undertaking the responsibility of burning buildings." In a private meeting they quickly got the reassurance they sought. According to the Board's minutes, "The government was willing and ready to support whatever measures [the Board deemed] necessary to put the city in a good sanitary condition." Among the measures explicitly endorsed were "detention camps" for people dislocated by the fire policy but still subject to quarantine. Though no one could predict the duration of the epidemic and no one knew for certain how many structures around the city would eventually have to be burned, the group agreed that construction should begin immediately on a detention camp capable of housing five hundred evacuees. And in all probability, they reluctantly agreed, "more than one" such camp should be anticipated. Dole then publicly reaffirmed the absolute power of the Board of Health for the duration of the plague crisis.[31]

Bolstered by the president's pronouncement, Emerson, Day, and Wood began to realize just how extraordinary their situation really was. Though they were nonelected public health officers, they were empowered—in the face of a world pandemic—to destroy private property; to incarcerate quarantined individuals in public camps; and ultimately to manage the affairs of the entire archipelago, public and private, in an absolute and essentially dictatorial fashion. To implement their decisions, they were deploying the militia, the police force, and the fire department. They were drawing huge amounts of money from the Hawaiian treasury, and their proposed actions would almost certainly require still-larger sums in the future. No checks or balances existed to counter the Board's decisions, regardless of how arbitrary or unnecessary they might appear to be. No meaningful routes of appeal lay open to those aggrieved by any of the Board's actions.

8

Public Health Policy and
the "Great Doctors' Meeting"

During the first week of January, Honolulu's death toll from plague began to rise slowly and steadily. On January 4, Board physicians confirmed four additional deaths, the largest number on a single day since the epidemic had reappeared at Christmas. That brought the total number of known plague deaths to nineteen. Even allowing for deaths concealed by friends and relatives, that figure was hardly astronomical, especially in comparison with death tolls reported in Canton, Hong Kong, or Bombay. But the pattern emerging in the first two weeks of the epidemic greatly frightened everyone in the city who was familiar with the way this current epidemic of bubonic plague had been harvesting its victims elsewhere.[1]

Most epidemic diseases that had attacked Hawaii in the past, like cholera in 1895, had typically done most of their killing in early waves that peaked quickly. Had that been the case with this pandemic, the fact that January's initial increases were relatively small might have been grounds for optimism. But public health officials all around the world had noted that the bubonic plague of the late 1890s typically killed relatively few people when it first appeared in a given area, then continued to kill in steadily accelerating numbers for the next several months, peaking long after its first appearance. The deaths of early January thus appeared ominous, the beginning of a relentlessly upward trend. Unless the plague could be stopped, the worst almost certainly lay ahead. Though modest by themselves, the rates of increase experienced in the first week of January would produce horrific totals if projected out several months. Western physicians, who read about these patterns in their medical journals, were especially frightened about the small but steady increases of early January.

All of the cases were occurring inside the quarantined district of Chinatown, and with each confirmed death came additional property condemnations, followed by additional burning orders and the need to house still more refugees in the city's quarantine camps. By the end of the first week of January, the men of the Honolulu fire department found themselves working from dawn to dusk, usually burning small or isolated structures in the morning and larger clusters of buildings in the afternoon. Emerson, Day, and Wood wondered privately in their daily meetings whether their fire policy might eventually result in the destruction of virtually everything inside the quarantined area if the epidemic continued to spread.

While the three physicians running Hawaii agonized about what might become of the quarantined district in the long run, others preferred not to wait and see. Rather than letting the epidemic become more virulent, they urged the medical triumvirate to strike first by preemptively torching the entire area in which the plague would almost certainly do its greatest damage—Chinatown. If the practical effect of burning confirmed plague sites seemed likely to result in a drawn-out, piecemeal destruction of the old slum anyway, why not get it over with quickly and stop the epidemic in its tracks?

To discuss that question, Emerson, Day, and Wood held a special meeting after dark on the evening of January 3. Dole himself came over to Board headquarters to take part in the discussion, accompanied by several of his closest advisors. Most of the latter leaned toward burning Chinatown in its entirety as quickly as possible, though they recognized the immense problems of dealing with the economic losses that would occur and the great difficulty of providing for the thousands of people who now lived in the buildings that would be destroyed. Still, the position of Judge George R. Carter was typical. Though Carter had been one of the three special agents who drafted the proposals for sanitizing Chinatown—the expensive proposals adopted only a few days earlier—Carter now privately urged his medical friends to accelerate the process by burning the entire area first. If you do so, he assured them, you will have "the support of the people." Lorrin Thurston, who had been overseeing the construction of new detention camps, told the three physicians that at least two thousand people could already be accommodated, and it would not take long to build more barracks.

Dole expressed reservations about the legality of wholesale preemptive burning. He had no difficulty with the policy of summary action where deaths had already occurred, but his legal background now made him think that formal notices for the abatement of nuisances should be served before torching properties not directly implicated in plague deaths. Attorney General Henry Cooper—the constitutional officer who presided over the Board of Health—conceded that the preemptive burning of Chinatown would be "a tremendous question to face," but he assured Dole and everyone else present that he could overcome any legal hurdles. In his view, Emerson, Day, and Wood should move aggressively to destroy the slum in the quickest and most expeditious manner they could.

Francis M. Hatch, a longtime government insider who had held several cabinet posts and who claimed to speak authoritatively for the city's leading American merchants, brought still more pressure when he told the three physicians that Honolulu's businessmen were increasingly concerned about the mounting "loss to the community from the suspension of trade"—and their own plummeting incomes. In Hatch's view, the white business community would support drastic measures of any sort, however costly and however arbitrary, as long as the measures promised a speedy end to the epidemic and an early restoration of international commerce, which they regarded as the lifeblood of the Hawaiian Republic. Backing that opinion, the *Commercial Advertiser*, the principal public voice of the merchant community, had already begun a steady drumbeat of editorial exhortations directed at the triumvirate, all of which argued that the preemptive destruction of the Chinatown slum was the step most likely to halt the expanding plague in the shortest possible time.[2]

Emerson, Day, and Wood felt squeezed. On the one hand, their New Year's policy had evoked threats of legal action from landlords and stirred the potential for civil unrest inside Chinatown; on the other hand, influential government insiders, powerful merchants, and increasingly strident editors were trying to bully them into even more radical action. It did not help that Emerson had been battling illness himself since before the New Year announcements. Writing to his sister the day after the special session with Dole and his advisors, he told her, "the war is still waging in and about China-town. I am not enough of a prophet to foresee when the end will be." Although he assured her that he was determined to fight on, he admitted that sometimes "I get very weary, and do not care whether 'school keeps or not.'"[3]

Assailed from all directions, the three physicians decided to stay the course they had set in the final days of 1899. At the conclusion of the special evening session, they formally resolved to continue burning buildings where cases of plague had been reliably confirmed, but they refused to order the preemptive destruction of Chinatown as a whole. The evening's discussion forced them, however, to recognize more clearly than ever both the probable need and the medical desirability of moving as many Chinatown residents as they could out of harm's way. With that in mind, the physicians drew an additional $250,000 from the Hawaiian treasury "for the expenses of the epidemic" and voted to begin construction of "barracks and accomodations [*sic*] for 5000 people." They also began to search for additional warehouses to store the growing piles of clothing, furniture, and household goods being removed from condemned buildings in Chinatown for fumigation and quarantine.[4]

Hawaii's attorney general was clearly irked at this outcome. The morning after Emerson, Day, and Wood rejected the hard line he advocated, Cooper officially resigned as president of the Board of Health, notwithstanding the constitutional provision that placed him in that position in the first place. He was spending so much time presiding as a figurehead over medical matters during the present crisis, he declared, that he was unable to function effectively as attorney general. As far as he was concerned, the doctors were henceforth completely on their own.

Undeterred, the three physicians themselves promptly elevated Clifford Wood to the presidency. Well organized, persuasive, and not easily pushed around, Wood was the obvious choice among the three and likely to be far more effective under the circumstances than either the ailing Emerson or the genial Day. No longer reporting even symbolically to the republic's attorney general, the triumvirate was now more independent than ever— particularly after Dole issued a personal statement of support for their current policies and his council of state not only acknowledged the election of Wood but reaffirmed the absolute authority of the Board of Health for the duration of the plague emergency.[5]

After electing Wood president, the doctors also accepted the resignation of L. D. Keliipio, who had been a civilian member of the Board for several years but had not attended a meeting since the fire policy was announced. Though little is known about Keliipio or why he resigned in the midst of the Board's reorganization, his withdrawal hinted at some disagreement, or at least nervousness, about being associated with the fire policy as it unfolded. Francis M. Hatch, who clearly had few qualms about burning anything and everything in Chinatown, accepted a presidential commission to take Keliipio's seat.[6]

From his first day on the job, Wood was an active president. To deal with the rising number of cases and to take some of the heaviest burdens off himself and his two colleagues, Wood ruled that any physician working under the direct authority of the Board, not just the Board physicians themselves, could officially pronounce a case to be plague. This greatly augmented the power and responsibility of the private physicians who were working on the front lines of the battle in such capacities as health inspectors and hospital attendants. Wood then formally extended the state of medical emergency and tightened the city's travel restrictions. The three physicians also imposed a ban on construction throughout the city, because they wanted to develop stronger sanitary codes for all new buildings and they needed all of the city's construction workers to help build quarantine camps. In yet another effort to explore alternatives or supplements to burning, Wood appointed Board member Smith a committee of one to consider the pluses and minuses of "disinfecting the ground in the infected district with sulphuric acid."[7]

To formally announce the new regime, Wood summoned the Chinese and Japanese consuls to a meeting at the Board of Health office. He told the consuls about the administrative changes and gave them a chance to voice any concerns they had about the fire policy so far. After Yang and Saito left, the three physicians went into executive session to discuss the continuing problem of concealed deaths, particularly among the Chinese. Another lengthy discussion ensued about whether or not to take some kind of action against those Chinese physicians who appeared to be complicit in that practice, but as before, the three Board doctors decided to avoid a direct confrontation with the Chinese traditionalists.[8]

Of more immediate interest to Emerson, Day, and Wood were prospects for improved relations between themselves and the Western traditionalists who belonged to the Hawaiian Medical Society. The December meeting of that society had publicly disavowed the Board's early quarantine actions and belittled the bacteriological evidence of plague. In the wake of that session, many Medical Society members had declined to serve as health inspectors, "stating they did not believe so far that the situation was so alarming as to call for extraordinary precautions." The incident strained longtime professional friendships and created a rift within the Western medical community of Honolulu. But the resurgence of plague since Christmas had validated both the triumvirate's early actions and the accuracy of Hoffman's initial conclusions, and as a result, some members of the Medical Society now seemed slightly embarrassed, anxious to abandon the skeptical stance they had assumed three weeks earlier.[9]

On Saturday, January 6, the Medical Society invited its members to another special meeting to reconsider the present situation. Current president of the Medical Society Charles B. Cooper (no relation to Attorney General Henry Cooper) quickly signaled the dramatic about-face of those who attended. In the evening's principal speech, Cooper declared that the Board's actions since Christmas had demonstrated that Emerson, Day, and Wood were now fully "deserving of the confidence of the people." Their willingness to use fire against the plague was singled out for special praise: "By no other act," Cooper asserted, "could the Board of Health have so completely" regained widespread support. Cooper's public endorsement carried added weight with the physicians assembled that night, since everyone present knew that Cooper was married to the daughter of John McGrew, the society's cantankerous founder, who had dominated the meeting three weeks earlier and openly attacked the Board's professional credibility.[10]

Other former critics pushed even further in defense of the triumvirate's right to act boldly. James H. Raymond, for example, who had belittled Hoffman's bacteriological conclusions and urged censure of the Board's actions at the Medical Society meeting three weeks before, now blithely asserted that "the question of the medical profession being the representative body of the people is a well-established fact," and it therefore followed that medical officers had a duty to force the city to do whatever was necessary for its own good. "The law of self-preservation" superceded any lawyerlike quibbling over formal lines of authority. Raymond personally favored the complete destruction of Chinatown, after which, following Kitasato, he thought the district should lie fallow for a year before being rebuilt to sanitary standards. In what the press reported to be "strong speeches," many other physicians, most of whom had previously refused to support the Board, spoke in a similar vein.[11]

Day—the ideal conciliator—replied on behalf of his Board colleagues. He began by acknowledging forthrightly that attendance was noticeably smaller at this meeting than it had been at the special session three weeks earlier. He and everyone else in the Western medical community knew that plenty of traditionalists had boycotted this meeting and still wished to remain at arms' length from the policies being pursued by the Board of Health. The Western physicians of Honolulu were far from unanimous in their approach to public health policy. Lest anyone miss that conclusion, the anti-Dole press went out of its way the next morning to undercut the Medical Society's about-face by observing pointedly that "most of the physicians in whom the people have confidence were conspicuous by their absence from the meeting."[12]

Even so, Day was delighted that the physicians who came to the meeting had decided to bury the hatchet. He reminded them that almost everyone present had been calling for many years for more extensive city sewers, better garbage incinerators, filtered water, burial reforms, and the "reconstruction" of slums like Chinatown. The plague crisis now offered an opportunity to achieve those goals as "emergency measures." "If we attempt to combat the plague by any other means," Day believed, "we shall have the same trouble as is experienced in Hongkong [*sic*], where the plague breaks out from year to year and is never entirely eradicated. Nothing but the most modern system of sanitation will do for us now." Hoffman then seconded the call for "radical measures" in Chinatown, which he described as "the dirtiest and most foul district I have ever seen."[13]

By stressing sanitation as a common ground for cooperation, Day's speech again revealed the ambiguous relationship between the new science of bacteriology and the long-standing traditions of earlier nineteenth-century public health. Bacteriologists believed that illnesses like plague arose neither from dangerous environmental conditions (as sanitationists had argued for more than a century) nor from problems within the body of its victims (as millennia of traditional physicians had assumed), but from specific microscopic agents that inflicted the disease. Even Cooper had conceded "the impartiality of the pestilence in smiting different races." Yet Day still placed his emerging ideas about bacteriology into a conceptual framework that regarded cleanliness as a cardinal element of public health.[14]

Physicians like Day and Hoffman no longer thought that filth produced diseases in and of itself, but suspected that foul conditions almost certainly harbored and sustained the disease-causing microbial agents that did produce diseases. International authorities supported that view, citing the fact that the vast majority of plague outbreaks in cities worldwide over the last five years had occurred in their least sanitary districts. Bacteriologists could thus comfortably continue to endorse traditional sanitation as a weapon in their fight against plague. And physicians like Cooper and Raymond, once convinced that plague was really present, found common ground with the Board in the form of familiar sanitary goals. Raymond made the point explicitly: "I think the question of unity in the medical profession on the subject of sanitation is one of the essentials of this meeting."[15]

At the end of the evening, the assembled physicians voted on a series of specific endorsements. Though a minority hoped that fumigation and disinfection might save parts of Chinatown, a majority of the physicians present joined the city's white editors and white merchants in urging that "all structures in the infected districts" be burned. The ground "where such buildings stood" should be cleared, disinfected, and left vacant for a year. Residents rendered homeless in this process should be furnished "sanitary habitations" at public expense. The physicians also strongly approved the Board's already-announced sanitary goals. Filtration systems sufficient to cleanse the entire Honolulu water supply should be installed. The city's small sewer system should be extended into all areas of the city not already served. And finally, the Board should force the city to launch a program of ongoing garbage destruction to prevent future accumulations of filth.[16]

What the pro-government press hailed as "The Great Doctors' Meeting" thus produced a paradoxical victory for Emerson, Day, and Wood. On the one hand, they regained the official support of the Medical Society, whose members had humiliated them just three weeks earlier. On the other hand, the same Western physicians who had previously told them they were going too far were now telling them they were not going far enough, and the resolutions passed by the Medical Society provided a professional imprimatur and medical rationalization for those already calling for the summary torching of Chinatown.

The *Commercial Advertiser* lost no time in hailing the Medical Society resolutions as confirmation of its earlier editorial admonitions regarding Chinatown and the plague. In bold capitals, it printed the Medical Society resolutions, and in strong editorials, that voice of the white commercial elite endorsed them in glowing terms. Reciting a litany of previous epidemics, all associated with Chinatown, the paper argued that Honolulu had "tolerated epidemics [there] too long." The time had come to do something about the conditions that had allowed those epidemics to gain their footholds and terrorize the city. Without forceful actions now, plague would hold on and recur into the future. "What of our tourists and our sugar cargoes then?"[17]

The *Hawaiian Gazette* had initially criticized Emerson, Day, and Wood for implementing policies that might end up "destroying thousands of dollars worth of property, breaking up hundreds of houses, and changing a prosperous section of the city into a smoking ruin." But now that the city's Medical Society had endorsed the complete incineration of Chinatown as "absolutely necessary if the plague is to be stamped out, . . . 'the greatest good to the greatest number' is the rule that must govern."

The following day, the Honolulu Chamber of Commerce, which had previously taken no formal stand on the fire policy, joined those howling for the preemptive burning of the quarantined district. In the chamber's view, the Chinatown slum, now certified by doctors as a dangerous affront to Honolulu's health, had to go.[18]

Representatives of Chinatown's large landowners and the district's residents themselves tried to counter the consensus emerging from white commercial interests and white medical professionals in favor of completely destroying the quarantined district. John F. Colburn, the outspoken counsel for several Chinatown property owners, drafted a public letter claiming that he and others like him had no particular quarrel with the Medical Society's sanitary recommendations, but strenuously opposed "that part of the resolutions adopted by the physicians at their meeting the other evening, which refers to the destruction of the buildings by fire in the infected districts, and the ground upon which such buildings stood to remain vacant for at least one year." Property owners were beginning to realize that they stood to lose not only their existing structures but also an additional year of income before being allowed to rebuild.[19]

Chinese vice-consul Gu Kim Fui, himself one of the city's leading merchants, arranged an interview with the *Commercial Advertiser* to urge caution. The Chinese merchants whom he represented hoped that the Board would hold to its stated policy of burning only those buildings where plague had been confirmed, not the entire Chinatown district. He also hoped that the value of condemned goods and buildings could be agreed upon and paid in advance. Provided that could be arranged, he had no objection to letting confirmed plague sites lay fallow for up to three years after burning. According to the *Advertiser*, "Mr. Goo [*sic*] Kim hastened to add that his remarks must not be construed as a complaint. Whatever the decision of the authorities may be, the Chinese will abide by it. . . . [T]hey fully realize that a half-hearted action will only prolong the strife and increase the loss to them in trade."[20]

Gu thus struck a balance between the militant opposition of many people inside Chinatown to the fire policy and the commercial interests of Chinese businessmen, which were not markedly different from those of American businessmen. Two days later, Consul Yang took a similar position. He no longer protested the use of fire at confirmed plague sites; he protested the hardships that the policy was imposing on the Chinese merchants affected by it. Clearly, both men had decided to accept the Board's targeted burns as better than complete destruction, and both men wanted to appear as cooperative as possible as they defended their interests.[21]

To increase pressure on Emerson, Day, and Wood, the Medical Society took the resolutions from their "great doctors' meeting" over the heads of the Board members and directly to President Dole. The press reported the doctors "unite[d] upon the most drastic proposal" to raze Chinatown completely, and the city's white newspapers strongly backed the Medical Society. Indeed, in their presentation to the council, the Medical Society delegation proposed not only burning the entire Chinatown district, treating the ground there with disinfecting chemicals, and allowing the area to lie exposed for a year to "sunlight and air," but also relocating the displaced population of the district to permanent settlements on higher ground elsewhere in the city. Toward that end, some of the physicians urged Dole to appropriate money expressly for the construction of new homes and businesses where Chinatown refugees could live permanently after their quarantine periods expired, rather than wasting funds on temporary resettlement camps.[22]

Among Dole's councilors, the Medical Society's presentation provoked a lively debate that mirrored similar discussions taking place throughout the city. In the minds of some, like the businessman Cecil Brown and the land developer W. C. Achi, financial issues were uppermost. They were nervous about opening the public treasury to any and all expenses involved in resettling the people and the businesses of Chinatown, either elsewhere in the city or in Chinatown. In the minds of others, like the wealthy patrician Peter Cushman Jones, humanitarian issues were uppermost. He claimed that everyone he talked to—from the members of his club to folks "down in the town"—agreed that the government had an obligation to help any victims from Chinatown. "We will not stand by," he was quoted as saying, "and see these people starving to death; we will go down in our pockets first." For still others, legal issues were uppermost. Was it right that an entire section of the city be obliterated on the orders of three physicians acting under emergency powers? In the end, Dole asked Attorney General Cooper to reiterate his official ruling that the Board of Health alone was absolutely in charge under the circumstances, and again refused to intervene.

For their part, Emerson, Day, and Wood continued to stand by the policy they had articulated and implemented on New Year's Eve. Through the first two weeks of January, the three physicians continued to condemn only those buildings where plague cases had been confirmed. Aware that many people in Honolulu favored more aggressive actions, Day conceded "that in the case of buildings which may or may not be considered dangerous to the public health the benefit of any doubt should go to the

people." Privately, new Board president Wood told Dole that the complete destruction of Chinatown appeared likely in the long run, since plague
deaths were continuing to occur at the rate of about one a day throughout
the Chinatown district, and the Board did not expect the epidemic to abate
anytime soon.[23]

Publicly, the three physicians also expanded the working definition of
a plague site by adopting the practice of condemning all of the buildings
in "close proximity to a place where a case of plague has occurred." Board
members were uneasy about that expansion and "deemed it advisable to
secure legal advic[e]" before making it. Yet once in effect, the expanded
definition increased the probability that most of the Chinatown district
would eventually be burned. Watching the number of displaced residents
rise exponentially with the growing size of plague sites, Emerson, Day,
and Wood on January 12 advised their ad hoc committee on detention
camps "to go ahead and erect sufficient buildings to hold, at least, five
thousand people from the infected places in the City of Honolulu." Though
no public announcements were made, the hiring of almost three hundred
carpenters detonated an explosion of rumors.[24]

Nonetheless, the Board's physicians remained committed to their original fire policy. As bacteriological believers, their goal was the destruction
of a specific bacterial enemy. Though they were inclined to believe that
pestis bacteria might establish themselves more easily in unsanitary areas
than in sanitary areas, they also recognized that not all unsanitary areas
harbored plague and that *pestis*, like many other types of bacteria, might
well be capable of sustaining themselves in perfectly sanitary environments,
such as in foodstuffs. Since Board members considered fire to be the only
tool at their disposal that was absolutely certain to destroy the enemy,
they had resolved to burn the enemy out. But unlike the sanitationists
around them, they aimed to burn only the enemy, not every place they
thought the enemy might be likely to attack.

Consequently, through the third week of January the Board of Health
continued to spare buildings that offered some promise of alternative disinfection by fumigation or other means, as they did on January 10, when
they exempted the Yee Wo building on Smith Street from an order to
burn the other structures in that block. They also responded favorably to
a request from several Chinese merchants that two Chinese representatives join the Board's team of property assessors. And even if they wanted
to begin burning more aggressively, Emerson, Day, and Wood realized
that first relocation camps had to be constructed and then systematic property appraisals had to be carried out; both of which took time. Finally,

since they were the government of the Hawaiian Islands, the three physicians could not irresponsibly create unmanageable situations: they had to maintain public safety and public order.[25]

Thus while a majority of the Medical Society's members, most English-language newspapers, and the city's white businessmen all urged a scorched-earth campaign in Chinatown, the ruling triumvirate of Emerson, Day, and Wood remained committed to a search-and-destroy mission, with Hoffman's microscope the means of detection and controlled burns the means of eradication.

9

Fighting with Fire

W ith plague deaths a daily occurrence in Honolulu through the first three weeks of January, the physicians on the Board of Health tried to keep their focus on Oahu. But because their emergency oversight included the entire Hawaiian archipelago, they also had to monitor events on the other islands, a task that brought them into direct conflict with panicky local officials. On Maui, Kauai, and Hawaii, residents unilaterally refused to recognize the Board's authority. Rather than take instructions from Honolulu, they preferred to isolate themselves and deal with any plague crises that might occur on their own. Officials on Kauai were resolutely turning all vessels away at gunpoint, whether cleared by health inspectors at Honolulu or not. The sheriff of Hawaii County, though technically under the command of the Board of Health in Honolulu, refused to allow a medical officer sent by Wood to come ashore at Hilo. When the re-buffed medical officer returned to Honolulu with that news, Emerson, Day, and Wood officially stripped the sheriff of all authority but still had to negotiate a settlement with Hilo's local citizens, who clearly agreed with their sheriff's position.[1]

Shipping agents and labor bosses lobbied constantly for exceptions to the embargoes placed on the movement of goods and people from island to island within the archipelago. Particularly irate were many of the white

American sugar planters on the outer islands, whose regular supply of labor had been interrupted indefinitely by the Board's travel rules. Since the vast majority of the plantation laborers being imported to Hawaii at this point were Japanese, and since many of the Japanese in Honolulu were awaiting jobs on the outer islands, where they would be not just clear of the epidemic but finally earning some money, the sugar barons and their lawyers joined Japanese labor contractors in a campaign of complaints to the Dole administration about the Board's absolute ban on Asian travel. The planters were, to say the least, rather ironic champions of Asian rights, yet another example of the complicated dynamics and strange bedfellows produced by the plague crisis.[2]

The three physicians found themselves besieged with a host of peripheral problems in Honolulu as well. Residents complained that garbage scow operators were not carrying potentially contaminated materials as far out to sea as the triumvirate had ordered. To catch the operators in the act, sixty-year-old Emerson rowed secretly out to the end of the harbor early one Sunday morning with a Hawaiian assistant, and the two of them witnessed the "discharging of garbage and refuse not more than 1/3 of a mile from the mouth of the channel." That scow operator was fired, but his successors did not do much better. Drifting debris and unpleasant odors became regular features along the city's waterfront, an unintended consequence of the cleanup programs underway in Chinatown.[3]

The collection and fumigation of personal possessions and commercial merchandise from contaminated areas consumed large amounts of time and money, since almost every detail of the process was regularly challenged by some party with a vested interest, many of whom retained the city's most influential law firms to back them up. Records had to be kept, buildings had to be commandeered as fumigation stations, and agents had to be paid to do the actual work. Those opposed to confiscation and fumigation circulated false rumors that owners would be billed for the service.[4]

As the number of deaths continued at a steady rate of roughly two a day, so did the number of additional plague sites that had to be burned. With each day's burnings, more people were rendered homeless and had to be relocated, accommodated, and temporarily incarcerated in the city's burgeoning quarantine camps. Upon arrival at the camps, the detainees were disinfected in special showers. Because they had been directly exposed to plague, they were forced to remain in the camps for three weeks, where they were closely observed every day for symptoms. Acceptable living quarters had to be built, sometimes by contractors and sometimes by residents, and this necessitated procurement of large amounts of lumber and hardware. Fresh water had to be located, then piped in and pumped to appropriate outlets. Such basic items as clothing, blankets, and furniture had to be provided, since all of the detainees' own possessions had been taken for fumigation and storage or already destroyed if they were deemed impossible to disinfect. And, of course, everyone had to be fed.[5]

Although the camps offered sanctuary for displaced persons at a safe remove from known plague sites, where the government provided essential services at public expense, the camps were neither voluntary nor altogether beneficent. Some of the camp directors tried hard to make the situations tolerable, and some Chinese and Japanese camp occupants wrote testimonials praising the efforts of individual camp administrators and expressing gratitude for the treatment they received. But people in the camps had been forced to surrender their possessions, give up their livelihoods, and accept the destruction of their dwelling places as the result of governmental policies in which they had no say whatsoever. Armed guards made sure they remained in the camps for the period of their quarantines. By the middle of January, the number of people confined in the Honolulu quarantine camps rose to over a thousand.[6]

In place of the ad hoc associations that had sprung up during the first quarantine, ethnic and religious groups from outside Chinatown now organized formal aid societies to help people who were displaced, interned, and later relocated as a result of the fires. These new organizations generally limited their assistance to their own kind. The Chinese Aid Society attended only to Chinese homeless; the Japanese Aid Society only to Japanese homeless; and the Hawaiian Aid Society only to Hawaiian homeless. The charter of the Japanese Society, for example, stated its purpose as helping to compensate for "damages sustained by fellow-countrymen in consequence of the sanitary fires." Church organizations likewise focused their attention principally on fellow religionists.[7]

Preexisting aid societies also came forward to help. Activities of the Ahahui Kikua Manawalea Hawaii [Hawaiian Relief Services Association] were typical. Originally founded during the cholera crisis to aid Hawaiians, this organization was popularly known as the Mothers' Relief Society, since it was headed by a team of Hawaiian and white women. On behalf of Hawaiians relocated to camps, the society organized clothing drives, inspected facilities, lobbied the Hawaiian aristocracy to provide supplemental resources for Hawaiians, and met directly with Board president Wood whenever they saw things that needed correcting.[8]

The various aid societies proved remarkably effective and well supported, primarily because most of the people living outside the quarantined district were more affluent—and hence in a better position to help others—than their ethnic counterparts inside Chinatown. Praise was universal for the work of the societies, which also arranged temporary school classes for interned children. Emerson, Day, and Wood strongly encouraged the work of the aid societies, met frequently with their representatives, almost invariably agreed to implement their suggestions, and afforded them a sort of semiofficial status.[9]

To help implement their policies elsewhere around Honolulu, the beleaguered physicians on the Board of Health somewhat reluctantly reactivated and expanded their previously authorized Citizens' Sanitary Commission. Behind that action lay the decision to resume twice-daily inspections of the entire city, not just of Chinatown. Emerson, Day, and Wood did not want a single plague case to escape notice, and they needed a constant flow of detailed information in order to react quickly wherever the bacilli struck. And despite some misgivings, the three physicians saw no realistic way to accomplish such extensive surveillance without a large volunteer force loyal to the government. Their principal misgiving stemmed from their realization that most members of their December medical posse had now become enthusiastic backers of the aggressive agenda advocated by the Medical Society, the English-language press, and the Chamber of Commerce, rather than the Board's own more selective approach. "As the Sanitary Commission expresses it," reported the *Gazette*, "'when in doubt, burn the house.'"[10]

As expected, the Board's lay inspectors pressed steadily for the destruction of all sites they deemed unclean, whether diseased or not. Surely it was no accident that most of the sites they brought to the attention of the Board were inhabited by Asians. J. P. Cooke of the Planters and Merchants Committee, which was closely allied with the Citizens' Sanitary Commission, warned Board president Wood that many Chinese and Japanese originally from Chinatown had relocated around the city between the two quarantine periods and were now overcrowding Asian enclaves all over Honolulu. If nothing was done to eliminate such situations, each of those areas had the potential to become "a menace to public health, in fact a minanature [*sic*] of Chinatown." Cooke had this information, he said, as the result "of good inspecting on the part of the Agents of the Board of Health." But the Board continued to insist upon bacteriological evidence of plague before ordering sanitary fires.[11]

Tension escalated to the point where the frustrated directors of the Citizens' Sanitary Commission, whose members now included the formidable Lorrin Thurston, went directly to President Dole and the Council of State—

as the Medical Society had done before them—in an effort to force the Board into more wholesale condemnations. Though all of the directors of the Citizens' Sanitary Commission were close personal friends and staunch political allies of the president, Dole again refused to intervene. The Board of Health's absolute authority remained intact, but relations became awkward, defensive, and at times downright confrontational between the Board's three physicians and the lay inspectors acting in their name.

By carrying out their duties in a heavy-handed fashion, Citizens' Sanitary Commission inspectors provoked ill will throughout the city, particularly among nonwhites. The Hawaiian-language press reported a procession of Hawaiians being "taken like prisoners" from condemned sites to the Kakaako camp by armed agents of the Citizens' Sanitary Commission. "There were also Japanese, Chinese, Gilbertese, Indians and others in the procession." Some had "tears streaming down their faces . . . as they reflected on the homes which were about to be destroyed by fire by the government." When they turned "their sad eyes and faces" toward a crowd of spectators, they saw "white men and women . . . taunting those being led off by the government guards." Hawaiians found such "reprehensible acts . . . sad and pitiful." "Those whose homes were taken and burned are like prisoners of war" in the hands of the Citizens' Sanitary Commission, concluded *Ke Aloha Aina*, when they should be treated instead as innocent refugees from the war against plague. "It is a ridiculous situation."[12]

Since they were supposed to monitor the ongoing health of every person residing in their assigned district, Citizens' Sanitary Commission inspectors had the right to enter homes and examine individuals twice a day. People being inspected complained of petty theft, insensitivity, invasions of privacy, and racial harassment. On his first day of service, one of the inspectors was indicted for attempted rape after he entered the home of "a respectable young white woman, demanded to 'inspect' the premises, and when in a room alone with her, assaulted her and tore her clothes." In his own defense, he claimed to have been too drunk to remember what he had done. No wonder that the Chinese protested loudly that many other inspectors had "little respect for Chinese womanhood." At one point, Citizens' Sanitary Commission agents had to be publicly reminded that "harsh treatment of women of whatever nationality will not be countenanced by any intelligent citizen."[13]

Hawaiians reported similar indignities inflicted by agents of the Citizens' Sanitary Commission. Everyone evacuated from a plague site was sent to a disinfection station prior to relocation in a quarantine camp. At the station, people had to surrender their personal effects, including jewelry and money, then strip for a mandatory medical inspection and a disinfecting shower. After that they were provided with fumigated clothing issued by the government. Sometimes as many as 250 people would be processed in this manner in a single morning.[14] Hawaiians resented the fact that white guards not only commandeered their valuables, which were not returned, but also "stay[ed] and watch[ed] the private parts of women" during the process. "And what's worse," reported *Ke Aloha Aina*, "is that some of the women are experiencing menstruation at the time, and are not able to shield or protect themselves from the orders of the guards, with their spectacles examining the private parts of these people. The wife of the president of the Board of Health would be treated better had she been among these Hawaiian women who are subjected to abuse. What are his policies regarding these lustful inspectors? We imagine that he would quickly order a halt if such things were happening to his wife. Can he not just as quickly put an end to the glaring of the inspectors at the privates of men and women and the seizure of their belongings?"[15]

Economic hardships followed closely behind personal indignities as sources of distress. Chinese and Japanese merchants inside Chinatown resented the seizure of suspect goods by Citizens' Sanitary Commission agents, particularly since individual inspectors had considerable discretion in what they decided to categorize as potentially suspect. In theory, owners would get their confiscated goods back after a period of warehouse storage and fumigation, but in practice all perishable items were effectively lost and durable merchandise was often damaged. And in the meantime, the merchants had nothing to sell. To make matters worse, "certain irresponsible people employed as guards and carriers" were blamed for the "plundering of goods" in storage. Both Chinese and Japanese businessmen suspected that their white competitors were taking advantage of these circumstances and happily pushing their friends on the Citizens' Sanitary Commission to implement the Board's ostensibly medical policies in ways that hurt Asian merchants.[16]

Japanese consul Saito Miki complained repeatedly to Emerson, Day, and Wood about other alleged abuses as well. According to reports reaching Saito, some of the Japanese commercial goods that were seized for storage or fumigation had not been disinfected at all, but simply hauled to a central spot, where they lay outside on the ground, unattended and vulnerable to rain and theft. And like the Hawaiians, Saito protested the behavior of Citizens' Sanitary Commission volunteers who administered the mandatory disinfecting stations. "At the time of disinfection, the Japanese are said to be rather ill treated by the guards and officials connected with the quarantine," Saito protested. "For example, they say that men and

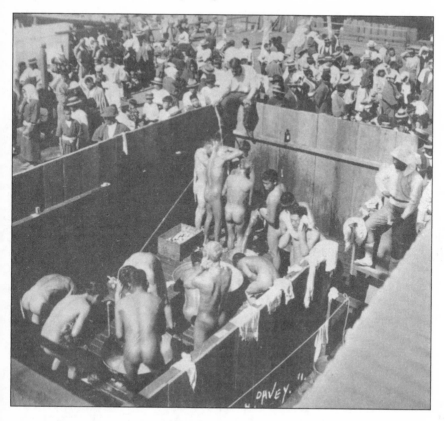

Japanese men receiving disinfection baths. Hawaii State Archives

women were all put into one line, entirely naked, and thus fumigated. Then they were driven along the street by the guards who had a stick in their hands as though they were driving sheep. The Japanese, even the lowest class, are not accustomed to this kind of treatment, and they can not endure it." Saito urged the doctors to intervene personally.[17]

In his reply, Wood denied the intentional destruction of any Japanese goods and denied "there been any ill treatment of the Japanese of any kind." On the basis of reports reaching him from physicians on the scene, Wood asserted that it was "utterly untrue that men and women have been put in one line naked at the time of disinfection. The men and women have been entirely separated at the time of giving the disinfecting baths." But he did concede that "some trouble has been made by a few Japanese men, keepers of, or residents at, the bagnios [brothels] of Pauahi Street. The respectable class of Japanese, however, have worked with the agents of the Board in the utmost harmony." President Wood and his two colleagues on the Board fully realized that the agents acting in their name were a mixed lot, some of whom no doubt thoroughly enjoyed playing the role of petty tyrant. To avoid future embarrassment, the three physicians quietly began hiring matrons to attend female refugees in the camps.[18]

The Board continued to meet every morning and almost every afternoon, seven days a week. Every day brought news of another death inside Chinatown; up to five people died on bad days. Hoffman, the Board's bacteriologist, performed autopsies virtually around the clock, and the city's refurbished crematorium was in nearly continuous use. Most of the victims were Chinese and Japanese; a few were Hawaiian. Some people in the city became convinced that *pestis* lived mainly in Asian foodstuffs, or could at least survive in Asian food and be spread when eaten. After all, with the exception of Ethel Johnson, people who ate Western foods were still unaffected by the epidemic, while those who died had eaten mostly Asian foods. And the papers all noted that Ethel had been eating Chinese candy she bought at an Asian market shortly before she came down with plague. So the Board had to spend a great deal of time debating whether or not to fumigate, destroy, or ban foods imported from Asia. The Board's first order of business, however, remained the ongoing condemnation of specific plague sites, as reported by Citizens' Sanitary Commission inspectors, confirmed by the Board's authorized physicians, and formally voted by Emerson, Day, and Wood personally.[19]

The fire department spent almost every day executing the Board's orders, usually running one or two days behind the formal condemnations. As a practical matter, burning specific sets of buildings, even burning separate blocks, was a difficult and dangerous task. The overwhelming majority of structures in Chinatown were wood, most were packed densely together, and many were quite flimsily constructed. Every fire had the potential to spread beyond its intended target, as accidental fires had regularly done in previous years, sometimes with disastrous results. The worst of those accidental conflagrations had occurred in 1886, when a runaway kitchen fire in a Chinese boardinghouse destroyed most of Chinatown below Beretania Street and triggered mob violence by Hawaiians against Chinese, whom the Hawaiians of the district blamed for their losses.[20]

To minimize the danger of fires spreading, the fire department calculated wind speed and direction, then ignited buildings only under specific conditions and always from particular angles. Once the fire was underway, the firefighters stood by with their hoses playing on nearby structures to prevent them from catching fire, and they dampened their target fires to keep them from burning too furiously to be safely contained. Embers lifted by updrafts were chased down and extinguished. "On all the surrounding buildings ... groups of Japanese and Chinese armed with brooms and shovels" typically gathered to help the fire department "prevent burning sparks from setting fire to their habitations."[21]

Honolulu had long been proud of its fire department. In advance of most cities its size, Honolulu had engaged full-time professional firefighters to staff the city's fire stations, including the so-called chemical engine station located near the center of Chinatown. As the station name implied, the Honolulu fire department kept up with the latest fire-fighting technology, in this case a large four-wheeled version of the soda-and-acid fire extinguishers that remained common throughout the United States into the late twentieth century. The city fathers had also invested in a brand-new steam pumper, dubbed Engine No. 1 by the men, that arrived in the islands only a few months before the plague. Trained volunteers, some of whom had organized themselves as ethnic associations, assisted the paid professionals when needed.

For their burning of plague sites, the firefighters received consistently high marks from the Board of Health, the city's newspapers, and outside observers. Many stories appeared under headlines like "Good Work of Firemen," and many editorials praised the ongoing efforts of the department. Chinese, Japanese, and Hawaiian spectators regularly applauded the skill with which the controlled burns were accomplished. When firemen successfully burned a meeting hall on Pauahi Street without even marring the brand-new Chinese-owned wood-frame lodging house right next to it, they received special commendations from residents of the neighborhood. Cooper quipped that the city's firefighters had become so good at this work that "they could go into a house and burn out one room without harming the remainder of the building."[22]

The fire chief of San Jose, California, who happened to be vacationing in Honolulu when the plague crisis struck, also had high praise for the ability of Chief James Hunt and his men in Honolulu to control the fires they set, especially under such difficult conditions. "It is a more trying test of Chief Hunt and his men to handle a deliberate destruction of property, than to simply drown out the ordinary fire," the visitor observed. He lauded Hunt for using the methods of "the best fire departments in the great cities." Ironically, the only hint of criticism directed at the fire department during the early weeks of January was an editorial urging Hunt's men not to douse their fires too quickly, lest a few plague bacteria somehow survive.[23]

Despite effective implementation of the fire policy, the epidemic contin-ued to produce daily deaths inside the quarantined zone. More ominously, the plague soon showed disturbing signs of breaking through the quaran-tine lines. On January 10, plague struck a national guardsman named Kauehoa, who had been patrolling the perimeter of the quarantined dis-trict, and Kauohi, one of the Board's temporary employees, who had been operating an excavating machine inside Chinatown to clean privies and re-move garbage. Both men were Hawaiian and both regularly returned each night to their homes outside the quarantined district. Both men died three days later. Two more Hawaiians living in different districts—and lacking any apparent contact with the quarantined zone—died the following day, as did a Chinese man inside the zone. The evident spread of the epidemic dismayed Emerson, Day, and Wood, who promptly ordered the four Ha-waiian death sites to be burned, the first such burnings outside Chinatown.[24]

On January 14, Honolulu's white residents opened their morning news-papers to the dreaded news that one of their own, forty-six-year-old Sarah Boardman, had apparently come down with plague. Boardman and her husband George, a high-ranking civil servant, lived with their niece in a comfortable suburban home in the Nuuanu Valley. Their personal doc-tor, a homeopath named George Augur, had called the Board of Health office seeking help with a grave case, and when Day and Wood took a carriage out to examine the case for themselves, they had almost immedi-ately diagnosed Boardman as suffering from plaque. They also learned that she had probably contracted plague at Jordan's dry goods store on Fort Street, where she was the art director. Jordan's had recently experi-enced an infestation of rats, and the two physicians assumed that the rats must somehow have carried the disease to a commercial section of Hono-lulu otherwise regarded as clean and prosperous. Two nurses were keep-ing watch over Sarah Boardman, but the physicians were not optimistic.[25]

President Wood immediately declared the Boardman house to be a plague site, notwithstanding its location in what the press called "one of the best residence sections" of Honolulu. Wood then ordered armed agents to remove the other members of the household to a guarded detention site. A veterinarian was summoned to chloroform the couple's eight prize pugs on the grounds that those valuable show dogs might also carry the bacteria. Pickets patrolled the house where Boardman lay critically ill, and Wood imposed a general quarantine across the lower section of the wealthy Nuuanu Valley.[26]

"The community was shocked beyond measure," reported the *Com-mercial Advertiser*. "The announcement of plague symptoms developing in Mrs. Boardman caused a feeling of apprehension to spread over the city." Unfounded rumors of additional cases "threw the city into a fever of excitement." Previously silent white citizens from Honolulu's upscale neighborhoods now began to speak out. E. F. Bishop, for example, appeared personally before the Board as the delegated representative of the Nuuanu Valley's residents. Those prominent and prosperous citizens strongly objected to the relocation of Boardman's family to a guarded detention center, and they vigorously protested the general quarantine imposed on their own neighborhood. But the Board held its ground.[27]

For two days, the daily papers anxiously kept track of Sarah Boardman's status in detailed front-page stories, and couriers kept Emerson, Day, and Wood informed of every development. She experienced a typically forceful first onslaught, accompanied by high fever and bodily pain, then slipped into semiconsciousness. The following day she seemed to improve, her fever receded, and her attendants experienced the cruel hope of recovery so characteristic of bubonic plague. But while Wood was presiding over the regular afternoon meeting with his colleagues on January 16, a courier entered the room and slipped a note from Augur under his hand. Wood stopped in midsentence, read the note, and grimaced. His expression "caused the remainder of the Board to fear the worst," and Wood somberly announced that Boardman had died ten minutes earlier. The assembled group then condemned her home to be burned as a plague site.

Sarah Boardman's death shocked the white community. Many whites had been wishfully maintaining their supposed immunity to plague, and some had been maintaining an almost blasé attitude toward the epidemic. Now, according to the press, they "finally came to the belief that steps should be taken by them to assist the Board of Health." In private session with President Dole and the Council of State, a discouraged Wood candidly reported the Board's failure to contain the epidemic within the boundaries of Chinatown and confessed his frustration at not knowing exactly how the quarantine lines had been breached. Boardman's case, he feared, promised to be merely the first of many more among Honolulu's Euro-Americans, and the Board's three physicians were bracing for a possible "panic"—his word—among the city's whites. "Then what is to be done?" Wood wondered aloud to the president.[28]

Through all of this, Emerson, Day, and Wood had been continuing to implement their fire policy with daily burnings wherever plague cases were confirmed. Prior to the demise of the four Hawaiians and Sarah Boardman, all of January's deaths had occurred in Chinatown, so all previous burnings had taken place there as well. The fire department had conducted its largest

burning yet on January 12, when it successfully incinerated an entire me-
dium-sized block on the eastern edge of Chinatown immediately adjacent
to the rest of the city. The following day the firemen burned an area known
as Union Square. On both occasions, "the streets were filled with people of
all races to watch the fires lit by the government." Commercial photographers recorded the events in black-and-white images, which they repro-
duced overnight and sold to the public the next day, despite criticism that
the circulation of such pictures in the United States could damage business
and discourage tourism. But the death of Sarah Boardman galvanized a fresh
round of rhetoric urging the peremptory eradication of the entire Chinatown
district.[29]

Editorial after editorial in the white press implored the Board to abandon its site-by-site policy and stamp out the principal locus of plague in
its entirety, before the epidemic had a chance to spread still farther afield.
Boardman's case "caused widespread consternation" and reminded Americans that "the plague does not always respect the white skin." The rat that
passed the disease to Boardman was almost certainly "a Chinatown refugee," and the rest of the city should no longer tolerate that font of death.
The time had come to stop "dilly-dallying" and stop "respecting the property of this or that owner or estate in Chinatown." The message was clear
and repeated daily: the "active manufactory of the bubonic plague" in our
city is Chinatown, and "we shall have millions of deadly germs [if that
district] . . . is not purified by fire." Emerson, Day, and Wood were admonished to "Abolish the plague spot, gentlemen of the Board of Health.
. . . The rotting spot must be burned out."[30]

The three physicians responded to the cresting wave of panic and pressure by promulgating stronger building and sanitary codes, closing all
schools and places of public amusement throughout the city, and aug-
menting the Citizens' Sanitary Commission. In a public meeting attended
by "about a hundred citizens," Wood authorized the commission to move
beyond daily observations and to conduct a thorough census of all persons
in the city, making a list of all illnesses, right down to sore throats. The
Board physicians further curtailed public transportation and forbade all
changes of residence throughout the city without their permission.

But the ruling triumvirate of Emerson, Day, and Wood refused to abandon the basic principle of burning only confirmed bacterial sites, however
broadly defined, even within Chinatown. Indeed, with the prospect of
additional cases popping up all around the city, that principle seemed more
important than ever. Carmichael, the United States Marine Hospital Service officer, commended the resolve of his three friends on the Honolulu

Board of Health. "People who become frightened" under circumstances like these "only make matters worse," he told the Citizens' Sanitary Commission. As a matter of fact, he quipped half-seriously, "it would be a really good thing" if all those people who were trying to stampede the Board into more extreme actions "could be accommodated with passports" and allowed to leave.[31]

Countering the extreme anti-Chinatown sentiment throughout the city, the Board physicians took steps in defense of the district. They formally recognized the appointment of F. M. Brooks, a leading white attorney, as official representative of the United Chinese Society, some of whose members had feared that Consul Yang might sell them out in exchange for preferred treatment of his own business allies. President Wood even authorized Brooks to attend the Board's regular meetings and speak for his clients. On the afternoon of January 19, the Board sent another clear signal by staying a preliminary order to burn Chung Kun Ai's City Mill. Overzealous inspectors from the Citizens' Sanitary Commission had reported City Mill to be rat infested, but Emerson, Day, and Wood accepted the arguments of Henry Holmes, Chung's white lawyer, who pointed out that a building still under construction could not yet be infested with rat nests, that no one had died at City Mill, and that, as a practical matter, the Board needed the mill to continue processing lumber to build facilities for the people displaced by other condemnations.[32]

Notwithstanding their firm responses, the deteriorating situation was beginning to strain the working relationship of the Board's three physicians, and for the first time since they assumed power together, the triumvirate disagreed over a major policy. The disagreement involved the promise they had earlier given Consul Yang that all Chinese commercial goods would be fumigated and stored if the merchants provided storage space. This process had become so tedious, expensive, and time consuming that Wood had come to the conclusion that it should be abandoned, particularly for perishable goods, which Wood considered the most likely to harbor bacteria and the most likely to lose their value in any event. Once Wood made up his mind, his friends knew that he would be hard to move. Even so, the politically savvy Emerson, a veteran of many dicey public health situations, and the affable Day, Wood's lifelong pal and medical partner, both demurred. For the time being at least, Emerson and Day blocked the president's desire to alter the Board's original promise to the Chinese businessmen.

Speaking "in very strong and impassioned language," Wood vented his frustration to representatives from the Council of State. The primary goal of the Board's policies, he argued, was the relocation of vulnerable humans away from plague sites, which could then be destroyed. But now, he said, "We feel that the plague is gaining on us; and that we are not throttling it as we should. We have not been able to remove the population [from diseased sections of Chinatown] as expeditiously as we would like." In his mind, the two prime reasons for the lack of progress were "the wasting [of] time and energy . . . handling . . . large amounts of merchandise" and the fact that the Board "had no place to put the people." Though under intense public pressure as the Board's president and point man, and more than a little annoyed with his closest colleagues, the strong-willed Wood eventually calmed down. When he did, the three physicians regrouped to continue their campaign against *pestis*.[33]

10

The Burning of Chinatown

Determined to maintain their policies intact, Emerson, Day, and Wood continued to condemn specific plague sites on a daily basis. The fire department, in turn, continued to execute controlled burns. On Saturday morning, January 20, Chief Hunt and his men prepared to incinerate a tangle of shacks in what was identified on the quarantine maps as block 15. The doctors had walked that block themselves on Tuesday afternoon and had returned to their office to formally condemn the shacks, when they learned that Sarah Boardman had died.[1]

Although the fire department had burned much larger buildings earlier in the week, Hunt took unusually strong precautions on Saturday morning because the condemned shacks were within a few hundred feet of Kaumakapili Church, the most visually prominent and revered landmark in the Chinatown district. The fire chief knew the story of how the building's patron, King Kalakaua, had personally rescued "the people's church" during the kitchen fire conflagration of 1886 by rushing to the scene and directing destruction of the buildings around it. The king's quick-witted actions on that occasion had created a fire break that saved the church, and since then the building had enjoyed near-mythic status. Hunt certainly did not want to be the one who lost it.[2]

Hunt ordered every member of his department to be present for this Saturday morning burn, and he had all four of the department's pumping engines placed in standby positions near the church. The chief and his assistants carefully assessed both the terrain and the configuration of the structures to be burned, calculated the direction of the morning's soft breeze, and decided exactly where to begin the fire. As usual at these sanitary burns, a crowd of Chinatown residents gathered to watch. Commercial photographers, who obtained special passes, steadied their tripods. The day's controlled burn was ignited at about 9:00 A.M.[3]

By all accounts, the fire began exactly as planned. Once well established and blazing vigorously, the flames started to move slowly away from the church, exactly as Hunt had anticipated, destroying the condemned shacks in an orderly manner as they advanced deliberately toward the hills above Chinatown. Suddenly, however, after about an hour, the morning's light breezes gave way to strong gusts coming powerfully down off the *pali* slopes that rose steeply behind the city. Such an abrupt shift of wind conditions, uncharacteristic for that time of day and that season, caught everyone by surprise. In a matter of minutes, the bellows-like downdrafts turned the planned fire back upon itself and transformed what had been an orderly burn into something resembling an open blast furnace, complete with a dangerous fountain of burning embers rising sixty feet into the air.

Given the speed with which all this happened and the force of the unexpected gusts, Hunt's men had no hope of damping the original fire. Instead, they concentrated their efforts on preventing its spread backward, especially in the direction of Kaumakapili. Engine No. 1, the new pumper, had already been stationed at a key post next to the church. The firefighters operating that engine maintained a steady soaking stream on the building, and for a brief period Hunt's men on the ground held the fire back. Overhead, however, one of the windblown embers lodged near the top of Kaumakapili's eastern spire and ignited the steeple. Hunt ordered his men to aim for the top of the steeple and to risk bursting their hoses if necessary, but none of the fire department's engines was capable of generating enough pressure to propel water up to the fire in the steeple. One heroic firefighter entered the church, climbed to the roof rafters, made his way along the beams, and chopped a hole to employ a chemical extinguisher on the steeple fire. But flames rushed through the hole against him. He barely managed to escape alive.

From the steeple, the fire worked back along the roofline and down into the main part of the building, where it ignited large piles of clothing brought to the church from previously condemned plague sites for fumigation and storage. Realizing that they could not save Kaumakapili, the firefighters redeployed downwind, toward the center of Chinatown, in an effort to save the next series of buildings across the street. As they did so, flames broke through the roof and walls of the church and ignited the surrounding shops and rooming houses. Horrified onlookers did their best to help the firemen shift positions by dragging hoses and hauling engines. Hawaiians in the crowd wept openly as their principal church became fully engulfed in flames. "On all sides could be heard the moaning and praying of the natives," reported a white observer who was busily documenting the events with his camera, "some chanting the hymns they had learned there, and inwardly blaming the white man for the trouble and destruction, and still hoping [the church] might be saved."[4]

With their support beams burned out from under them, Kaumakapili's bells crashed through the church's burning roof to the sanctuary below, sounding "their own dirge, like the harmonious death-wail of some many-voiced living creature," according to an eyewitness. Many of the fervently religious people watching all this must have thought they were witnessing

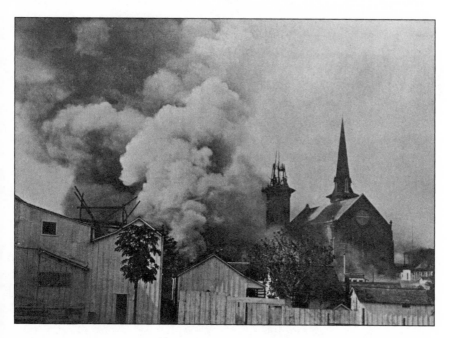

The great fire begins: buildings behind Kaumakapili burning out of control and one steeple partly destroyed. Hawaii State Archives

something akin to an Old Testament visitation. Honolulu's favorite church had become, for all intents and purposes, an avenging bonfire from which a steady spew of sparks and glowing gleeds rode the unrelenting gusts toward thatched roofs and wooden buildings elsewhere in the district. The well-fanned embers, in turn, ignited countless spot fires, often some distance from the church itself and frequently in unexpected or inaccessible places. Though people throughout the area tried their best to extinguish the spot fires, many of the small outbreaks were nearly impossible to reach.[5]

As the *pali* winds widened the leading edge of the fire and fanned it toward the center of Chinatown, flames jumped across the street from Kaumakapili Church to another set of densely packed wooden buildings and impassable alleys. That complex ignited quickly, and soon became a second major source of floating embers. Trapped on Beretania Street between the two largest conflagrations, Engine No. 1, the newly acquired pride of the Honolulu Fire Department, began to blister from the heat. With their clothes beginning to smolder, the exhausted firefighters operating that engine finally had to abandon the pumper to the flames or be enveloped themselves. As it was, they were saved only when bystanders dragged them to safety. Their comrades carried on as best they could from a safer distance, but the situation was clearly out of control.

By the time Emerson, Day, and Wood heard about the crisis and rushed over from their regular morning meeting downtown, Kaumakapili Church was fully enveloped and all of the buildings in three adjoining blocks were blazing uncontrollably. The intense heat created updrafts that constantly replenished a huge cloud of flaming debris and glowing embers. Some of the updrafts were strong enough to float flaming straw mattresses several yards above the ground. The firefighters continuously redeployed out ahead of the wind-driven fire, trying desperately to check its advance downward toward the harbor. They threw as much water as their remaining engines could pump at some of the threatened buildings, and dynamited others in an effort to create gaps too wide for the fire to jump. But they could not impede the expanding fire front.

Chinese, Japanese, and Hawaiian residents of the district tore down buildings with axes and ropes and tried to remove combustible materials from the path of the fire. They also attempted to stamp out small side fires wherever they could safely reach them. But burning debris continued to waft onto roofs in the middle of interior structures, where no one could get at them, and the intense heat prevented close actions of any sort against the fire's advancing face. Members of the fire department made a con-

The Burning of Chinatown

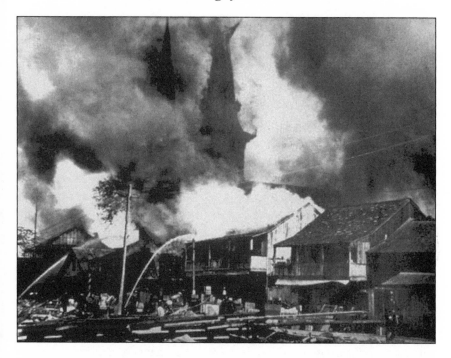

Fire spreading across the street from Kaumakapili Church. Hawaii State Archives

certed stand in defense of their own Chinatown district station, known as
the chemical engine house, but were unable to save it. By noon, the inferno was essentially on its own, spreading wherever the midday gusts and
free-drifting embers impelled it. As the fire raged on, volunteers entered
the quarantined district and conducted door-to-door searches, lest anyone become trapped inside buildings.

While the downhill drafts pushed the main fire through the center of
Chinatown toward Honolulu harbor, the original planned fire had resumed its intended course up the gentle slope above Kaumakapili Church.
But no fire equipment remained to check its advance when it reached its
intended limits, so it inched slowly onward against the downdrafts, toward a street of commercial buildings that included a warehouse known
to contain substantial amounts of kerosene and a large supply of fireworks
ready for Chinese New Year, only nine days away. Though people could
easily track the almost stately progression of the original fire beyond its
intended terminus, they had no direct source of water available and could
do nothing to stop it.

Residents of the area, mostly Japanese and Hawaiian, organized the evacuation of their neighborhood as the up-slope edge of the deliberately advancing fire approached the warehouse. An initial explosion of kerosene drums lifted the roof completely off the warehouse and distributed still more burning debris around the area, where it ignited additional smaller fires. Secondary explosions ripped through crates of fireworks for half an hour before the warehouse finally collapsed in a pile of charred rubble. Several Japanese and Hawaiian families barely escaped a runaway line of flames that accelerated unexpectedly from the vicinity of the warehouse down an alley and through their shanties. Other Japanese and Hawaiian residents selflessly destroyed their own homes to create a firebreak that successfully prevented the flames from continuing on up the slope toward the stylish residences of the Nuuanu Valley.

Downwind from the center of the fire, below the smoldering remains of Kaumakapili Church, firefighters continued to do what little they could, while retreating foot by foot toward the ocean. "Volunteers passed buckets of water to the men at the hose nozzle, drenching them constantly, but . . . the heat was so terrific that the steam arose in white clouds from the men." Many observers noted later that most of the firefighters were blistered across their faces and hands; some were burned quite badly. Volunteers and residents shuttled infants, the elderly, and infirm people to safe areas on the edges of Chinatown, where their cries of terror, in the words of a Chinese witness, "shocked the earth." Two Chinese men who were unconscious from opium smoking were rescued just before their building collapsed upon them.[6]

To the spontaneous applause of onlookers, electric company linemen risked their own lives to climb poles and bring potentially lethal live wires safely to ground, lest the writhing and melting coils fall among the increasingly desperate crowds rushing through the streets. Shortly thereafter, Hawaiian Electric cut all current to downtown Honolulu, adding to the chaos of the afternoon by disabling electric water pumps, leaving the telephone company without switchboards, and darkening offices; but the decision probably saved lives inside Chinatown.[7]

By 2:30 the strong winds that continued to gust down the face of the volcanic slopes above Honolulu had spread the fire several blocks to the east and west of Kaumakapili Church and driven its leading edge five blocks south, to within a few hundred feet of the city's main harbor. There the fire threatened the principal shipping wharves of this international trading city, as well as several small factories, various warehouses, City Mill, and the Honolulu Iron Works. Next to City Mill a large supply of re-

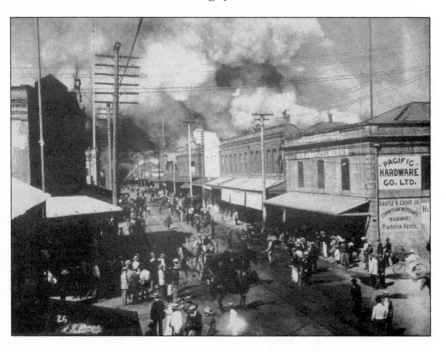

View from a downtown building as Chinatown burns in the background, with refugees trickling out. Hawaii State Archives

cently cut lumber, which had been neatly stacked beside the wharves, caught fire and burned quickly. That fire, in turn, ignited the main building of City Mill, which the three physicians had spared on appeal only the day before. Members of the Board, who were standing by as this took place, issued an ad hoc order to volunteers and firefighters to spare no effort in trying to save City Mill because they realized they would need it more than ever in order to build relocation camps. But the mill burned completely. When Chung Kun Ai reached the scene, he wept. His newly purchased machinery—not yet even paid for—was twisted and molten, resembling puddles of "lava stone," and he assumed he was ruined.[8]

A group of citizen volunteers and firefighters tried but failed to save the Murray Carriage Factory adjacent to City Mill, but fortunately none of the dozens of cans of oil inside the factory exploded. When the fire then began to turn along the waterfront toward the commercial heart of the city, white merchants in the crowds that had massed along Nuuanu Street began hiring bystanders to help them evacuate their own merchandise to safer ground. Frantic ship captains, fearful of the steady shower of burning embers landing on their decks, and realizing that the main fire would soon reach the shoreline, desperately worked to disentangle the lines that held their vessels to the city's wharves, so they could move to the safety of open water.

To reach the center of the city, the fire would have to pass through the buildings and grounds of the Honolulu Iron Works, something the firefighters and all of the Iron Works' two hundred employees were bent upon preventing. The factory had some key advantages over other structures in the Chinatown area. The outer buildings of the Iron Works were brick, providing the rest of the plant with something of a fire-retardant barricade. Before the fire reached them, the Iron Works' employees removed most combustible materials from the grounds. And most importantly, the Iron Works stood immediately adjacent to the seawall. In addition to the fire department's hose lines, employee-manned bucket brigades could help defend major structures, and waterborne fire-fighting equipment could be deployed.

Out in the harbor were two working ships with fire-fighting equipment on board, the U.S.S. *Iroquois* and U.S.S. *Eleu*. The city's small harbor dredge was towed away from the seawall, making room for the two larger vessels to pick their way against the parade of retreating ships and position themselves close to the seawall. The *Eleu* tried to keep the lumber mill fire from spreading, while the *Iroquois* began pumping heavy streams of water into the Iron Works compound, thoroughly soaking its major buildings. So powerful were the beams of water that onlookers felt them rock the buildings' foundations. Combined with the continuing efforts of the land-based firefighters and employee bucket brigades, these ships finally helped halt the great Chinatown fire at the edge of the Honolulu Iron Works. As the sun went down, the fire was burning itself out, the Iron Works were intact, and the rest of downtown Honolulu was out of danger.

For the residents of the burned over district, the day had been almost unbelievably terrifying, and the great Chinatown fire would disrupt their lives to an extent they could only begin to imagine that evening. Most of the residents in the vicinity of Kaumakapili Church, where the original fire had broken out of control, were Japanese and Hawaiian. These "frantic and, at first, terror-stricken people . . . rushed wildly up one street and down another." Even in the midst of this "tempest of excitement," however, they took great care to move the old and the infirm to safe places. Before the flames arrived, some attempted to lower furniture from second-story windows, while others tried to drag goods to safe places. But their efforts merely cluttered the already chaotic streets. For most people, the fire spread too rapidly and the heat was too intense for an orderly evacuation. They simply ran for their lives, abandoning their material goods to the hissing flames. "The condition of general misery and pandemonium in the area," remembered one of the Japanese caught up in the action, "made it seem just like a war zone."[9]

A crowd of mostly Japanese residents eventually began to congregate near a bridge that carried Kukui Street across the stream that defined the western edge of Chinatown. Since the district was already under quarantine, guards had been routinely stationed at the Kukui Bridge for the past several weeks. The guards who were on duty when the fire went out of control quickly concluded that they would not be able to block the increasing numbers of panicky refugees by themselves and sent word requesting militia reinforcements.

The request for reinforcements along the quarantine lines, according to white reporters on the scene, "gave the impression downtown that a riot was in progress, and citizens and military guards went to the scene on the double-quick." The city police captain positioned his substantial force of Hawaiian officers along strategic Nuuanu Street, where they blocked access into Honolulu's downtown business center to the east. Those officers were "armed to the teeth." Ordinary citizens, mostly white, also joined in, spontaneously arming themselves "with sticks, pick handles and pickets torn hastily from fences." An eyewitness remembered men from all over the city gathering "fire arms of all kinds, axe-helves, pick-handles, base-ball bats, and pickets, *anything* at hand that might serve as a weapon." This "pickhandle brigade," something between a vigilante mob and an ad hoc posse defending the public health, assembled around the boundaries of the burning district, determined to prevent the dispersal of a potentially plague-carrying population throughout the city. As a result, the desperate residents of Chinatown found themselves facing an inferno behind them and a hostile civilian militia massing all around them.[10]

As a growing number of hastily armed citizens from around the city arrived to bolster the quarantine lines, the potential for lethal violence escalated rapidly. The press had reported only the previous day that "the sale of small arms to Asiatics" had been unprecedented since the plague crisis began. Hoping to prevent a disaster, Consul Saito and his associates from the Japanese Aid Society rushed to the tense and confused scene on Kukui Street. Saito's entourage was immediately allowed to pass through the guard lines into the upper end of the burning district, where the consul moved among his countryman calmly reassuring residents that the

Board of Health was not out to exterminate them. Saito and his associates succeeded in preventing what could easily have become a deadly clash at the Kukui Bridge, then turned to restoring general order among Chinatown's stunned Japanese residents. They quickly established emergency relief and information stations, marked by "white flags with the red cross upon one and the Japanese flag symbol upon the other, [which] the people rallied to."[11]

Once the initial confrontations were defused, the residents of upper Chinatown were "allowed more liberty," and they settled down along the northern edge of the quarantine district to watch with resignation the relentless destruction of their homes and possessions. A large gathering of citizens from elsewhere around the city assembled above them on the slopes of the Punchbowl Hill to do the same. Most of the latter were women and children, since the vast majority of Honolulu's adult males had headed toward the fire to see what they might do.[12]

By the time the fire burned itself out that night, Chinatown's Japanese residents had lost all of their living quarters and seventy-six other establishments, including their neighborhood temples, churches, theaters, warehouses, factories, retail stores, grocery stores, offices, candy stores, and photography shops. Among the few things salvaged from the Japanese section of Chinatown that day were a printing press and a typesetting machine from the offices of the *Hawaii Shimpo*. With the help of the white sanitary inspector who had been monitoring that block under the quarantine, the *Hawaii Shimpo*'s assistant editor managed to drag the two pieces of equipment across Nuuanu Street, where they were retrieved by Japanese outside the quarantined district and stored in a Japanese school until the editor could begin publishing again.[13]

The situation was less calm in the central and lower sections of the district, where the fire moved faster and destroyed property more quickly than it had farther up-slope. As the fire encompassed block after block, thousands of predominantly Chinese residents of the area poured out into the streets to escape. They were, in the words of a spectator that day, "more or less terror-stricken, not knowing where they might go, what they should do, or what, in fact, was coming next." Even those with advanced warning barely had time to gather precious items; those taken by surprise left with nothing more than the clothes they were wearing. A few residents reentered buildings whose roofs were already on fire in desperate attempts to reclaim valuables, but they were largely unsuccessful. For lack of a safe place to store anything, most goods pulled from burning buildings had to be abandoned in the streets, only to be consumed there by the superheated fireballs bowling toward the harbor.[14]

According to an eyewitness reporter, "The frenzy of the Chinese and Japanese residents was pitiful to observe. They fled to the streets, lugging away at bundles too heavy for a man to ordinarily carry, but the keen excitement of the moment gave them the strength of two men. Women with strained eyes and tears rolling down their cheeks clung to little children and babes, in wild excitement, searching everywhere to find a place of safety. Few carried more than a change of clothing for their babies. . . . Every one was making a supreme effort to flee from the fire-fiend that destroyed their homes and household goods."[15]

Kong Tai Heong, Li Khai Fai's wife, who from the outset of the plague crisis had sided with her husband and the bacteriologists on the Board of Health, remembered the day of the fire in vivid metaphors. "The trees became live torches of flames!" she told her daughter decades later. "The roofs of the homes flashed red with flames and blazed crackling into the streets with hellfire! The streets crackled with the blaze and seethed with the hellfire . . . and shrieking cries, cries of people in terror!" She also recalled a darker side of the chaotic situation: "Some there were [among the Chinese themselves] who remembered only to loot and steal." Several press reports corroborated her memory of looting, which left a legacy of ill will within Honolulu's Chinese community for decades.[16]

Some wealthy Chinese merchants were reported to have lost thousands of dollars in gold to robbers who knew where it was hidden and took advantage of the chaos to move it. Residents caught one Chinese man setting fire to a building near the corner of Maunakea Street and King Street, where a store owned by Sing Chang was rumored to contain over eight thousand dollars in coins. The man was turned over to the quarantine guards and escaped mobbing by his fellow countrymen only because he was so "crazed with excitement" that his actions could plausibly be attributed to "temporary insanity." Several observers independently reported seeing Chinese residents deliberately igniting their own homes "in expectation of obtaining heavy damages from the Government." Though some of those incendiary efforts were temporarily extinguished by other people, the larger fire soon engulfed them anyway.[17]

Most of the district's Chinese residents congregated on King Street, which became "a dense mass of humanity" in the blocks beyond reach of the fire. Deeply and legitimately suspicious of the Dole administration from the early days of the Hawaiian Republic, and well aware of the public pressure to burn Chinatown in its entirety as quickly as possible, many Chinese believed that the day's fire was intentional, "that the Board of Health had purposely burnt their houses over their heads." The combination of fear and rage they experienced would be difficult to imagine. According to one eyewitness, "rebellious spirits among them urged a rush on the guards." Some Chinese were armed with handguns, and others nearly launched a full-scale riot by suggesting that the sound of exploding kerosene and oil containers elsewhere in the burning district was actually the sound of militiamen shooting people who were trying to escape the flames. "At this juncture," in the words of a Chinese resident in the midst of the crowd, "excitement was high and there was imminent danger of bloodshed."[18]

The threat of bloodshed was heightened by the presence of thousands of citizens now forming a thick human fence between the residents of the quarantined zone and downtown Honolulu. Mostly "men and boys," they were continuing to run from all parts of the city toward the great fire, and they were continuing to "arm themselves with every imaginable kind of weapon. Baseball bats and pick-helves were notably conspicuous, but in the volunteer army could [also] be seen . . . iron bars, hatchets, an occasional meat axe." The Chinese residents of Chinatown, already traumatized and furious, faced "a strong military guard . . . and . . . a line of citizens standing in reserve," determined to shield the city center.[19]

Chinese consul Yang moved among the crowds on King Street urging calm, but he was less effective with his politically and socially divided constituency than the Japanese consul had been with his more united constituency at the upper end of Chinatown. Early reports gave Yang some credit for maintaining order, but later reports accused him of spending most of his energy harassing government representatives on the scene and trying unsuccessfully to exact terms and concessions on behalf of Chinese businessmen from Emerson, Day, and Wood, who had neither the time nor the inclination to address such things in the middle of such an emergency. The three physicians were livid with the Chinese consul.

Fortunately, Yang was soon joined by Vice-Consul Gu, who had been visiting displaced Chinese in the Kalihi detention camp that Saturday morning when something from the direction of Chinatown caught his eye. Seeing flames above the steeples of Kaumakapili and "fire reaching the sky," Gu immediately bolted from the camp and joined thousands of others rushing toward the suddenly towering clouds of smoke. "There were crowds everywhere in town," he remembered. "Every street was packed." When he reached the guard line, Gu found a friend among the officers who recognized him and granted him permission to enter the quarantined zone. Once inside, Gu met hastily with various officials from the Dole administration who were also arriving on the scene, then began efforts to prevent mob violence. His first step was perhaps his most crucial: he persuaded the line of outside guards to pull back, in order to convince the desperate refugees that they would not be attacked. Gu then persuaded Yang to begin preparing for an orderly evacuation while he remained among the crowds for reassurance.[20]

The Chinese Aid Society came forward with food, water, and reassurances that helped Gu and others begin to defuse the situation. Members of the Board of Health, President Dole, and many of the leading members of the American elite also moved among the crowds, making clear through translators that everyone would be cared for if they maintained order. The refugees would have to remain under quarantine, but the government would find accommodations for them and provide everything they needed at public expense. Several authorities, including Dole himself, also repeatedly assured the victims that they would be compensated for their losses. As a result, according to one of the Chinese refugees, "the people of Chinatown subdued their rising tendency to do violence" and accepted "the representations of the authorities."[21]

Emerson, Day, and Wood, meeting in emergency session, ordered the release of anyone already in a quarantine camp who had not been exposed to a case of plague since January 11, freeing up nearly a thousand spaces for what the three physicians initially estimated to be approximately six thousand refugees. The Board physicians commandeered boxcars and public grounds, and empowered ad hoc citizen committees with the task of finding secure and habitable spaces around the city. The volunteer committees quickly obtained use of the capacious Kawaiahao Church, where the physicians started sending the first refugees by midafternoon. By late afternoon, while the fire burned itself out behind them, processions of Chinese, Japanese, and Hawaiians began to make their way from the quarantined zone down King Street through the city, where guardsmen and armed volunteers formed a human corridor that funneled the newly homeless toward makeshift lodgings.[22]

The evacuation and relocation of the fire victims went far more smoothly than anyone dared hope. A few of the refugees still urged an attack on the citizen guards who lined the route of exodus from Chinatown to the Kawaiahao Church and the nearby Iolani Palace grounds, but none was

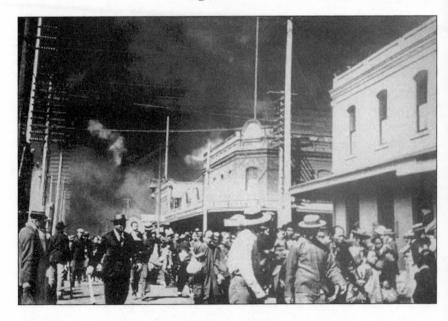

Exodus from Chinatown. Note the Chinese carrying bundles and the men on the left carrying axe handles. Hawaii State Archives

made and no one tried to escape the cordon of troopers and citizens. A few of the citizen guards "brandished clubs" at the frightened refugees, but apparently no blows were delivered. In the apt phrasing of the *Friend*, "the situation was most critical and dangerous, as well as moving to sympathy and compassion." Even an openly racist observer—he did not like the "hordes of filthy Japanese and Chinese" who brought to Hawaii their "peculiarly Eastern sins, crimes, vices, disease, and deaths"—noted that "A good many of these people were not coolies but of a better class, and in the haste and pressure were rather roughly handled, I fear; but no deeds of wanton cruelty were seen." "Where there are carriages without horses," noticed another eyewitness, "white men are taking the places of animals and pulling along small footed Chinese women and their babes or old and infirm people of all nationalities."[23]

We "were not in the least bit unruly," recalled one of the refugees, "and properly obeyed the orders of authorities. The authorities for their part did their best to provide relief." Photographs of the forced march out of Chinatown depicted a stunned and resigned population of refugees, many of whom were undoubtedly in various degrees of shock. Most of the faces that looked up at the photographer as they passed were, in the photographer's words, "patient and submissive." Newspaper reporters noted that "[m]any a mother, as she led her children along between the throngs of people, had tear bedimmed eyes," and the refugees were seen "casting frequent glances back at the red tongues licking up their homes." Hungry, thirsty, afraid, the victims were confronted by armed strangers who did not speak their language and feared them as the agents of bubonic plague. They were completely destitute to a degree they could not have imagined when they awoke that morning, and their future prospects were grim indeed.[24]

Eyewitnesses watched the painful steps of older women with bound feet, the struggles of people trying to drag salvaged possessions or paralyzed companions along with them, the bewilderment of children clutching household pets they had rescued from the fire, and the weeping of Hawaiians who clung to their guitars for solace. One white matron described the shock that people like herself experienced when they saw the refugees, not fully realizing "that Honolulu had a population such as that which passed between guards to the church." She felt intense sympathy for "the sorry crowd of sufferers" and noted that they were "perfectly submissive. The clubs [in the hands of the ad hoc citizen guards] were quite useless." The English-language press universally described the refugees in somewhat exotic but genuinely sympathetic terms, and editors universally urged the other four-fifths of Honolulu's population to mobilize in support of the victims.[25]

By late afternoon, observers estimated that 1,780 Chinese, 1,025 Japanese, and 1,000 Hawaiians had been successfully transferred to the Kawaiahao Church grounds, and at least another 500 people, mostly women and children, were inside the church itself. Armed civilians patrolled the perimeter of the churchyard, determined to prevent the "panic stricken mass of humanity" from "disseminat[ing] through the city the germs of plague from their unsanitary and infected abodes." Facing "perhaps the most distressing and dangerous condition with which the citizens of Honolulu have ever had to cope," Emerson, Day, and Wood requested help from the American military. The local commander, despite standing orders to keep his forces confined and away from any exposure to the plague, granted the Board's emergency request. Around 5:00 P.M. U.S. Army troops arrived at the church grounds and cleared the area of citizen guards, armed volunteers, and curious onlookers. This effectively ended the threat of civil unrest and freed the Board's relief committees to begin redirecting various refugee groups to other sites.[26]

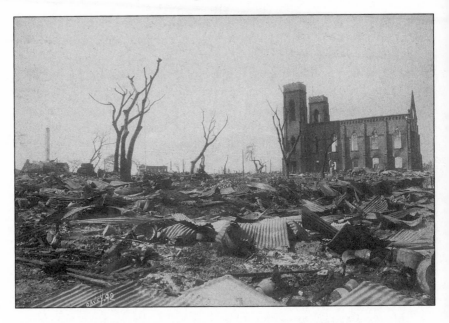

Ruins of Kaumakapili Church the morning after the fire. This photo was taken from a point just above the corner of Beretania and Nuuanu streets. Hawaii State Archives

Most of the Hawaiian refugees were sent to the empress dowager's property, to buildings controlled by Prince Kalanianaole, or to the Boys' Brigade headquarters behind Dole's executive office building. At all of those sites, the Hawaiian Aid Society dispersed poi and tried to restore morale. More than a thousand Japanese were sent to the Drill Shed grounds, also part of the executive office complex. A local businessman donated the use of a warehouse that accommodated 250 more people, and the Society for the Relief of the Destitute accommodated 500 others in buildings they had acquired along South Street. By nightfall, as the smoldering remains of Chinatown threw "a lurid glare" across Honolulu, "every quarantined person from the burned district had been provided with shelter and food." Miraculously, not one life had been lost during the fire. But for thousands of Chinatown residents, the day had been one of trauma and ruin, a day they would never forget, a day that would pass into Hawaiian lore.[27]

Curious sightseers came back the following day to survey the results of the fire. What had been a densely developed and heavily populated area roughly equal in size to twenty-five city blocks was now completely devastated. "It was hard," reported the press, "even for a person perfectly

The Burning of Chinatown

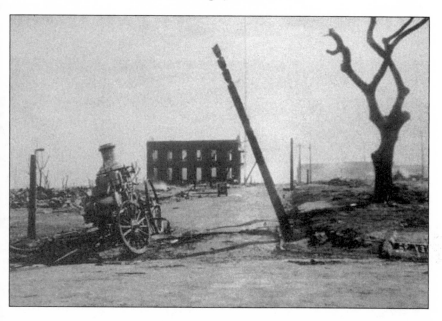

A burned-out fire engine and the shell of the Chinatown fire station. The station had been at the corner of Maunakea and Pauahi streets. Hawaii State Archives

acquainted with Chinatown, to pick out the places where various buildings [had] stood." The gutted brick shells of only five structures remained standing in what was otherwise a sixty-acre field of charred debris. The largest of those shells, the front facade of the Kaumakapili Church, would eventually have to be pulled down for safety. Intense heat had melted anything made of metal, even cooking pots. Sections of the ground had been baked to near-ceramic hardness. Strewn among the debris were over fifty safes, some open and empty, others intact. The latter were dragged to a central location where owners would be allowed to claim them.

Businessmen speculated that property losses from the fire easily exceeded $3 million, a sum that dwarfed any previous property loss in Hawaiian history—and no one knew how, or even whether, those losses would be compensated. In terms of material destruction, Honolulu had never experienced anything close to the great fire of January 20, 1900. Even under the best of circumstances, such a catastrophe would be difficult to address. But as Emerson, Day, and Wood recognized all too clearly, these were not the best of circumstances. Honolulu still had an epidemic of bubonic plague on its hands, which might now spread farther and faster than ever before.[28]

11

Detention Camps

After staying up all night directing emergency operations, Emerson, Day, and Wood reassembled at Board headquarters to assess the situation on the morning of January 21. Though the problems they faced were immense, they shared a bittersweet sense of relief. Roughly six thousand people had been evacuated from the burning district with no loss of life. Even more remarkably, no serious violence had occurred, despite the fact that the refugees, some of whom were armed, had lost absolutely everything in a fire that smelled to many of them like some sort of plot, probably hatched by white businessmen. Though traumatized and victimized, the vast majority of the refugees had gone along with the doctors' provisional orders, avoided confrontation with the ad hoc citizen guards who massed to hem them in, accepted the support provided by ethnic aid societies, and cooperated with the representatives of foreign governments.

Nor did the population outside the Chinatown district panic. Honolulu citizens of all races outside the quarantine zone had spontaneously armed themselves in an almost symbolic gesture of self-defense, and they had formed human barricades to channel the exodus from Chinatown to Kawaiahao Church. But no one struck a violent blow; no one made scapegoats of the refugees. That behavior too was remarkable, especially since the racist assumptions of whites in the crowd had been fanned for a week preceding the fire by editorials and letters in the English-language newspapers asserting that Mrs. Boardman's death was a harbinger of what lay ahead if the foul forces of the Chinatown slum were loosed in the city. The paper most friendly to the government later learned that many whites had refused to join the human cordon at all, and it chastised them as fainthearted. Honolulu's large population of Hawaiians also withheld any resentment they felt toward the Chinese and Japanese of Chinatown, even though they too blamed Asians for bringing bubonic plague into their city.[1]

Grateful for the rather amazing calm, the doctors acquiesced in the rapid withdrawal of the U.S. troops they had requested the previous afternoon. Carmichael and the American commander had violated their standing orders by letting those troops leave their base in the first place, so they were anxious to retrieve the soldiers as quickly as possible, hoping fervently that none of them would come down with plague as a result of their foray into the city. But Emerson, Day, and Wood were taking no chances around the refugee camps. They replaced the federal troops with regular shifts of Hawaiian Republic national guardsmen, some of whom were trained as sharpshooters.

While the plight of the refugees and the enormous questions surrounding their future occupied the immediate attention of nearly everyone in Honolulu after the fire, the three physicians dared not lose sight of the reason why they were still in charge of the Hawaiian Islands: the presence of plague. Indeed, the week preceding the fire had been the deadliest to date. Fifteen people had died, bringing the total to more than forty in the three weeks since the return of plague at the end of December.[2]

Publicly, Wood expressed the physicians' hope that the Chinatown fire might turn out to be a blessing in disguise. "Providence or somebody else had stepped in" to achieve something they had despaired of accomplishing so effectively: the safe removal of everyone from the most dangerous plague district in the city and the prompt destruction of virtually all of the goods and animals of that district that might be harboring bacteria. He offered reassurance to the rest of the city that there was "no great danger" from the refugees themselves, since they would be in quarantine for three weeks, and because plague seldom "communicated from person to person." And he "wanted to impress" upon everyone in Honolulu "that it was not people but localities that were dangerous, and to a minor extent the belongings of infected people." Surely the fire posed unprecedented civic challenges, but it might also provide the city with an unprecedented break in the battle against *pestis*. Wood did not want to lose that momentum.[3]

Consequently, that same day, the Board of Health met with representatives of the Citizens' Sanitary Commission and the Council of State to reaffirm their confidence in the policy of burning plague sites, despite what had happened the day before. In private session, the physicians on the Board received from Dole and Thurston the strong reaffirmation they sought. Thurston in particular agreed with Wood that the great fire, by obliterating what was far and away the largest and most dangerous source of plague, had presented the city with a unique opportunity to stop the epidemic once and for all by isolating and eliminating any remaining hot spots of disease. To forestall any crises of authority, President Dole reiterated publicly that "the Board of Health was [still] running the Government," and all "other executive members of the Government were . . . ready to back it up in any and every necessary measure."[4]

To signal their return to routine, the three physicians ordered the immediate resumption of close daily inspections and the submission of health

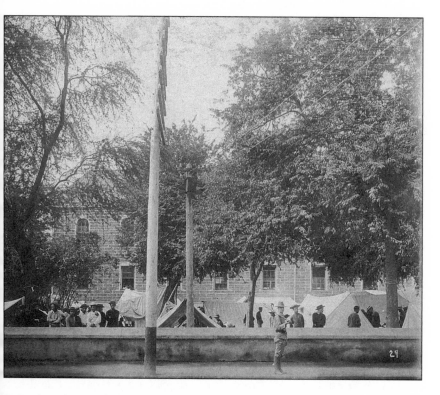

Refugees under guard outside Kawaiahao Church. Hawaii State Archives

reports on absolutely every person in the city. To help implement the renewed push, Thurston persuaded most of the city's white businessmen to suspend normal activities for ten days so that their employees, white and nonwhite, would be available to maintain the new inspection schedules. Emerson, Day, and Wood tried to make clear to their agents that they agreed with Dole's stated opinion that "no distinction should be made between nationalities" in the implementation of those close inspections: every individual of every race in every neighborhood would be rigorously monitored.[5]

With public order restored and their absolute authority reconfirmed, the Board's three physicians resumed their ongoing assessments of reported plague sites, some of which had not been consumed in the Chinatown fire. The fire department also resumed its targeted burns just two days after the Chinatown debacle, when it carried out the earlier order to destroy the Boardman property and a group of previously condemned buildings on the edge of Chinatown. Included in those fires were all of the Boardman furniture, the family's grand piano (even though Sarah Boardman had apparently never played it), and a "rare collection of curios."[6]

By January 26, all of the people initially assembled at the Kawaiahao Church on the night of the great fire had been relocated to more permanent detention centers, and the church itself had been thoroughly cleaned and disinfected. In just four days, volunteers acting under the Board's supervision had constructed scores of rough barracks at the city's principal quarantine camps. The barracks at the Drill Shed site accommodated about 1,200 people, the majority of whom were Japanese. Barracks at the greatly expanded Kalihi beach site became home to almost 5,000 people, some 1,500 of whom had already been at Kalihi due to evacuations and burnings before January 20. The majority of the people at Kalihi were Chinese, though some Hawaiians and many Japanese were there as well. Roughly 1,000 people thought to have been directly exposed to plague sites were transferred to the so-called Kerosene Warehouse site. That group included over 500 Hawaiians, over 300 Chinese, and slightly fewer than 200 Japanese. Along with approximately 700 people confined elsewhere, the Board found itself holding over 7,000 people in detention camps during the fourth week of January, or about one out of six residents of Honolulu.[7]

The process of camp assignment did not go seamlessly. A bold group of 248 Chinese men, for example, fearful that the Americans were sending them to death camps, initially refused internment at Kalihi and threatened to resist relocation by force. But Consul Yang persuaded them that the Americans would keep their word to provide food and housing, so the potential rebels agreed to divide themselves into groups of ten to help oversee an orderly distribution of the provisions rather than fight. A smaller group of Chinese men had to be forcibly restrained from tearing down relocation tents; a number of families that were accidentally separated in the confusion of the relocation process had to be reunited; and two babies were born to refugee women during the relocation process. But for the most part, the process went more smoothly than anticipated.[8]

To manage everyday affairs and most routine matters inside the various detention camps, the physicians on the Board of Health appointed camp committees for each site. To handle their increasingly complicated and now greatly enlarged fiscal operations, the doctors appointed an ad hoc Finance Committee comprised of Honolulu businessmen to advise them on such things as construction contracts and labor costs. They did not give the businessmen independent discretion, however, insisting instead that they themselves would make all final decisions. The triumvirate knew they were already under suspicion as pawns of the white commercial elites and did not want to feed those suspicions by giving free financial rein to the businessmen.

The new committees attended to such practical, though essential and expensive, matters as drilling an artesian well to provide the large Kalihi camp with a reliable source of fresh water. The Bishop Estate, the large holding company that owned the land where the Kalihi barracks had been built, agreed to pay for half the cost of the well, since the estate would benefit in the long run. But such seemingly straightforward and mutually beneficial measures nonetheless involved detailed negotiations, substantial amounts of time, a good deal of patience, and the commitment of public funds. In the case of the artesian well, the process was also complicated by years of bickering between the estate's trustees and the physicians on the Board, who publicly accused each other of disregarding or mishandling their prior responsibilities under the city's health codes. Similar issues were multiplied a thousand times as incident after incident and problem after problem arose day after day in camp after camp.[9]

All of the people displaced by the great fire of January 20 had to be fed, clothed, and generally cared for. With no time to think in advance about what they might need or what they might save, they were even worse off than those displaced by the earlier, smaller, and more systematically conducted evacuations. Some of the new refugees required medical attention, and all of them needed to be closely monitored during the next twenty days for signs of plague. So Emerson, Day, and Wood appointed other doctors to help oversee each of the major detention camps. To prepare

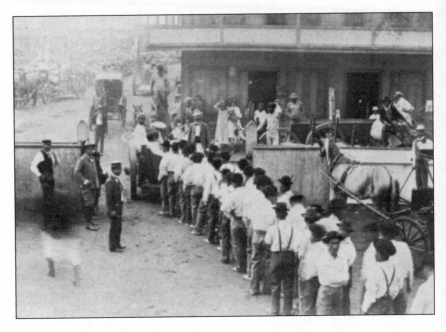

Refugees being taken to detention camps. They are dressed alike in government-issued clothing. Hawaii State Archives

food, camp directors employed some of Honolulu's top chefs, most of whom were out of work while the city's restaurants remained closed.[10]

Volunteers throughout the city began to collect household goods for distribution in the camps, while churches and other relief organizations redoubled their clothing and sewing drives. Wealthy whites donated thousands of dollars to the Chinese, Japanese, and Hawaiian relief funds that had been organized earlier in the month. The Board of Health also opened a donation center next to its own office, where people could deposit useful items that the physicians would then send to whichever camp was most in need at any given time. Literally tons of food, clothing, and miscellaneous goods quickly began to arrive.[11]

The huge outpouring of charitable support drew glowing reports from the Honolulu press. Swelled with civic pride, the city's most prominent pro-government editor publicly doubted that any American metropolis could have done as well as Honolulu in the wake of the great fire. In some ways, he may have been right. Looking back six months later, Carmichael reported to his Marine Hospital Service superiors in Washington that "all of the citizens united in a common cause; there was no bickering, and a more devoted, self-sacrificing community I have never seen." "Many of the most prominent citizens," he continued, "acted as sanitary inspectors, and all stood ready to help the authorities with their time and money in the fight against the plague."[12]

From inside the camps, the situation looked far less rosy. Some detainees, for example, regarded the city's charity as little more than hypocrisy: "This is like taking an arrow and wounding a man from a distance and then secretly go[ing] up to dress his wounds and soothe his pain in order to receive his thanks," wrote one of them, quoting an old Chinese parable. Letters written to the English-language press by irate Chinese detainees also continued to allege a conscious intent behind the burning of Chinatown. In vague terms, they warned of reprisal and retribution, perhaps when China rose again to world power or when the perpetrators of the great fire faced their God in the life hereafter.[13]

Vice-Consul Gu Kim Fui, who was allowed free access to his countrymen in the camps, formally protested overcrowding. At the Kalihi camp, Gu reported as many as twenty-five people sharing a room, and he complained that clothes and blankets were being held in storerooms rather than passed out to the needy. Trouble also arose over the health care of detainees. The Board allowed traditional Chinese physicians to visit their patients in the camps, provided they did not prescribe anything without the permission of a Board-appointed physician. When one of the traditional healers provided herbals on his own, his pass was revoked. Wood's position on the subject was unambiguous: "as long as the people were at the camp," he declared, they "[would be] under the Board of Health physicians."[14]

Other Chinese refugees took the less bellicose, but still sharply critical position articulated in a public letter from the chairman of a group calling itself the Chinese Citizens' Committee. Reprinted in the English-language dailies, the letter blamed the Board of Health for allowing the world pandemic to get through their protective screens in the first place, and then for failing to insist upon sufficient precautions when they ordered the burning of specific sites. The Chinese Citizens' Committee rightly reminded the people of Honolulu that the Chinese consul and vice-consul had repeatedly warned Emerson, Day, and Wood that many of Chinatown's buildings were dangerously close together, and hence difficult to destroy separately. Less than a week before the great fire, the Chinese consul had written formally to the government suggesting that wooden buildings be torn down and then burned, rather than burned in place, "thereby lessening the dangers to adjoining buildings." But their advice went unheeded, and as a result many of their compatriots had now lost everything. The Chinese Citizens' Committee realized that "what is done cannot be undone," and they appreciated "the kindly intention and expression of sympathy from a great many of the residents of Honolulu." But they also began what would become a steady drumbeat in favor of "a speedy and just settlement." Ongoing demands from the Chinese consul eventually grew so numerous that the English-language press reminded him publicly that he represented a weak government with little international influence and warned him that he risked alienating the general population if he did not desist.[15]

Though they did not openly rebel, most of the Chinese refugees forced into the detention camps by the great fire refused to cooperate with the Board's internal oversight committees. They declined construction jobs, regularly protested their conditions, insisted on the right to reestablish opium-smoking facilities in the camps, and generally signaled their unwillingness to help make the best of what they regarded as a fundamentally flawed policy. In the Kalihi camp, such protest actions were reported to be consciously organized under the tacit direction of Ah Hee, the proprietor of an up-and-coming carpentry shop on the Chinatown side of Nuuanu Street that was destroyed in the great fire.[16]

As the Japanese and Hawaiians had done earlier, the Chinese also complained bitterly about the humiliation of the camp's disinfecting procedures. Physical hardships were bad enough, they lamented, but "nothing compared to the shame, the black, black shame . . . brought upon our women, our wives, the mothers of our children! . . . forced to stand naked, stark naked in the streets for the white devils to see, for the whole world to see!" Vice-Consul Gu went over the heads of the Board and complained directly to Dole himself about just such an incident. According to Gu's informants, a Board-appointed physician was administering "antiseptics to bathe Chinese, Japanese, and native Hawaiian" women in the Kalihi camp, when some of the Chinese women, particularly those "who had bound feet or were shy," objected. The physician thereupon ordered "managerial personnel [i.e., ordinary camp guards, not medical people] . . . to take off their clothes by force." Dole promised an investigation, but the Board-appointed physician who gave the order, according to Gu, managed to co-opt Consul Yang, who reported back to Dole that he could find "no evidence of mistreatment of Chinese women." Gu felt the doctor should have been placed on probation, and the women involved in the incident wanted Vice-Consul Gu to sue the physician, Consul Yang's frustrating behavior notwithstanding. But the bathing procedures were changed the next day to provide more privacy and remove civilian guards, so Gu decided to drop the matter. The three physicians also arranged for Kong Tai Heong, Li Khai Fai's physician wife, to attend future disinfecting baths of Chinese women.[17]

For the incarcerated Chinese, the New Year that began January 29 was especially depressing. Gu was unsuccessful in attempts to have earlier refugees released, since they had now been reexposed to the victims of the great fire. In terms that echoed the tone of white comments a month before, when Christmas brought not joy but the return of bubonic plague, a Chinese internee commented to a reporter that the great fire might prove to have been good for everyone in the long run if it ended the plague, but it was "awfully sad" in the short run. "And none of you can understand our feeling on this our great holiday." Ironically, the holiday began the Year of the Rat.[18]

In addition to the lingering enmity they felt toward Honolulu's rulers, the Chinese refugees inside the camps remained deeply riven among themselves. Low-ranking laborers blamed their plight upon the wealthy Chinese merchants for whom they worked, believing that the latter should have been looking out for them rather than their businesses over the previous several months. Even before the great fire, they pointed out, wealthy Chinese families had persuaded the Board to let them foot the bill for special quarantine camps of their own, where they paid out of pocket for special services and accommodations that the Board was not providing in the ordinary camps. Poor Chinese women resented their more affluent counterparts whose bound feet made them "perfect nuisances" in the eyes of those who had to care for them under camp conditions.[19]

Preexisting political animosities also worsened in the camps. Qing dynasty loyalists and overseas reformers blamed each other for putting Honolulu's Chinese in such a vulnerable position in the first place, politically riven with no powerful government back home to defend their rights. Detainees established rival political societies inside the camps. Fights broke out among them over jurisdictions within the camps, and those Chinese opposed to the emperor back home had their allies outside the camps send separate delegations to the Hawaiian Foreign Office to apologize for the actions of Consul Yang and to protest the fact that they had to be represented by him. This further strained the already uneasy relationship between Yang, who had been sent from Beijing, and Gu, the moderate Honolulu-based vice-consul. The Board's camp committees eventually divided the Chinese refugees formally into separate blocs to help maintain order.[20]

Plague and Fire

Li Khai Fai and Kong Tai Heong, the husband-and-wife physicians who had worked with Emerson, Day, and Wood from the outset of the plague crisis, experienced the intense hatreds inside the camps in very personal ways. From the time they helped report the first cases of plague in Chinatown, Li and Kong realized that many of their countrymen would criticize them and the other Chinese doctors who sided with them, like Tong San Kai, the director of the Wai Wah Yee Yuen hospital. But Li, Kong, and Tong continued to regard the attitudes of their traditional colleagues as backward, superstitious, and ultimately dangerous to their own patients, so they had pushed self-consciously ahead with their pro-Western activities, Li quite aggressively.

Now inside the Kalihi detention camp, where he and his family had been swept up with thousands of other Chinatown residents on the day of the great fire, Li became both a convenient human lightning rod for the frustration of his traditional rivals and a traitor in the eyes of many of the Chinese who had lost everything in the fire. "Curse him, that bastard of the white devils!" they shouted as they passed his barracks in the detention camp. "Let us never forget this 20th day of January, let us never forget that this man of our own race was the one who brought disgrace upon us!" They felt they had been ruined "because of that devil Dr. Li."[21]

For Li, Kong, and their two small children, life at Kalihi was thus doubly miserable. Like all of the others, they were trying to make do with almost nothing in a temporary camp under armed guard; but they were also singled out as the agents of everybody else's misfortune. As Kong later remembered in poignantly poetic language:

> The days in camp crawled slowly, as though the centuries had come to live with us. And even though our friends were constant and our spirits strong, still the hours of our existence seemed heavy, as though hung with the leaden weights of time, motionless as the waters of a lotus pond gone stagnant with the scum of rotting life. But the sun was bright in its sky each day, and the hours of the night were quiet with the utter exhaustion of the spirit grown limp and almost lifeless with the nothingness of nothing. Every day, I kept washing and washing everything which I could find that needed washing, even though I was allotted only one bucket of water a day. . . . Every day, after the day's work of uncertain living slid into the night's endurance of fitful dreaming, [we] tried to take care of the sick ones in the camp, in spite of the jeers of [a rival] and his friends, in spite of the melancholy of their voices counting and recounting over and over again their misfortunes, disagreements and dislikes.[22]

Detention Camps

Though Li Khai Fai and Kong Tai Heong continued to live in Honolulu for more than fifty years after the great fire, many of their old opponents and professional rivals never forgave them for their actions during the plague crisis. Despite their large multiracial medical practices and their well-earned reputations as prominent civic reformers, Li and Kong continued to endure accusations that their betrayal of ethnic solidarity had led directly to the disaster of the great fire being visited upon their countrymen. After Li's death in 1954, gothic legends arose about his personally having thrown sick countrymen alive into fires ordered by the Dole administration for the purpose of eliminating Asians. Even today, oral traditions among some Honolulu Chinese still refer to Li as "Doctor Death."[23]

Less overt dissension appeared among the Japanese and Hawaiian refugees, most of whom apparently decided to make the best of the situation.

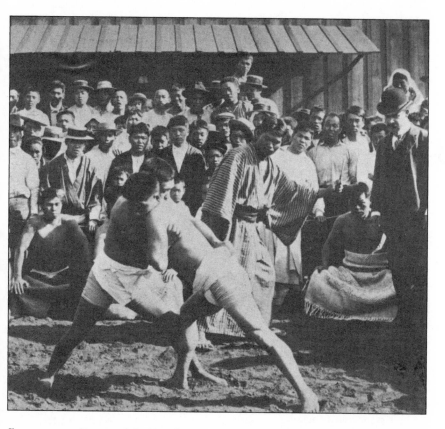

Japanese wrestling match inside a detention camp. Hawaii State Archives

Japanese consul Saito remained a steady and calming influence, both among the Japanese refugees and in the eyes of the Board of Health. Some tension arose over health care, and at least one of the Board's physicians was assaulted by a Japanese man who resented the physician's attempt to examine a sick Japanese woman. Camp managers also had trouble with criminal gangs among the Japanese refugees, some of whom had been running gambling and prostitution rings in the Chinatown district before they too had been swept up with the rest of the population on the day of the great fire. When the gangs started fighting among themselves and preying on fellow Japanese detainees, national guardsmen were called in to arrest them. Ordinary Japanese helped the Board's camp managers construct a jail on the Kalihi grounds to confine the worst of the criminals.[24]

For the most part, however, the Japanese camps ran smoothly. Refugees later recalled that clothing, blankets, and even mosquito netting were supplied by the authorities, and most Japanese considered the camps "fundamentally civil" under the circumstances. Food supplies in the Japanese sectors, which were supplemented by the Japanese Aid Society, proved more than ample. Once men and women were separated, the Japanese actively welcomed the "anti-septic" baths and "scrubbed one another in great glee; . . . as they realized it was for their own benefit." Consul Saito offered prizes for wrestling contests, and children received impromptu schooling with the help of donated educational supplies.[25]

These strategies largely worked, especially at the Drill Shed camp. The English-language press generally portrayed Japanese internees as models of admirable behavior and lauded their industriousness, cleanliness, high morale, and cheerful order. Emerson, Day, and Wood granted "a Committee of Ladies" in Honolulu official permission "to establish a home for fallen women who wish to lead better lives" at the Kalihi camp, in order to help provide for Japanese prostitutes. Life in the camps remained exceedingly tedious, of course, and at least one young Japanese man—alone, sick, and depressed—hanged himself. At the time of his suicide, he was under surveillance as a potential plague case, though an autopsy revealed that he did not have the disease. Still, when Emerson, Day, and Wood granted special permission for a prominent white business manager to spend a night at the Drill Shed camp to see for himself just how well or how poorly his seventy-five Asian employees were being treated there, the business manager found conditions surprisingly comfortable. "The Board of Health and the men working for them certainly deserve the greatest credit," the visitor believed, for what they were able to provide under the circumstances.[26]

Detention Camps

Like most of the other Japanese from Chinatown, Soga Yasutaro, assistant editor of the *Hawaii Shimpo*, also ended up in the Kalihi camp. There he roomed with his senior editor and the senior editor's wife, and together they all made do "in what seemed like a hut with a thousand other people." Bored, restless, and no doubt uneasy with the awkward housing arrangement, Soga slipped through the police lines one night, jumped the quarantine barrier, and headed for the home of friends elsewhere in the city. He eventually hid out "in the dirty, little upstairs room in Ishimura's Cook School on Kukui Street," along with the printing equipment his white friend had helped him salvage on the day of the fire. In less than a week, by acting as if he had never been in quarantine in the first place, he was able to resume his activities in support of Honolulu's Japanese leaders. He played a major role in organizing the Provisional Japanese Council to address the needs of the hundreds of homeless Japanese still inside the camps.[27]

Affairs seem to have run most smoothly among Hawaiian refugees, who were fewer in number than the Chinese or Japanese. From the beginning of the fire policy, most displaced Hawaiians had been quarantined in separate camp facilities, many of which were specially constructed on sites owned by various members of Hawaii's deposed royal family, and the hundreds of Hawaiians driven from Chinatown by the great fire joined those already interned in those separate camps. Partly owing to their favorable living conditions, refugees in the Hawaiian detention camps were generally well fed and seem to have maintained good morale. The Hawaiian Aid Society raised large amounts of money on their behalf. Hawaiians who corresponded directly with the Board of Health about various problems were answered promptly in their own language.[28]

Hawaiians certainly did voice their disgust with what had happened and with the hardships visited upon them by the government. In particular they grieved the great loss—actual and symbolic—of their Kaumakapili Church, and they placed the blame for its destruction squarely upon "the ineptness of the Board of Health." They also grieved the loss of so many other landmarks of "Old Honolulu," and they protested the treatment of Hawaiians who had lived in the Chinatown area for generations. Only the "cruel and merciless" would allow dignified elderly women, who had lost all of their family mementos, to be "herded up like horses and mules and corralled." But even the most inveterate antigovernment editors ultimately accepted the medical rationale that lay behind the tragic incident. *Ke Aloha Aina* urged Honolulu's Hawaiians to remain calm, keep the peace, and go after individual wrongdoers—like guards who committed robbery—rather than attempt to revolt.[29]

One of the most difficult problems the three physicians faced in the weeks after the fire was the tension that resulted from having to house large numbers of various racial and cultural groups together in the same detention camps. Japanese refugees did not want to be intermingled with Chinese refugees, whom they regarded as backward and dirty. The Chinese, who were already subdivided among themselves along political and social lines, felt the same way regarding the Japanese. Hawaiians from the outset had sent "committees to meet with the Board of Health and the government to ask them to separate all Hawaiians . . . so that they are not mixed together with the Chinese and Japanese." George Boardman's Euro-Hawaiian ancestry had provoked a flap on the eve of the great fire over where and with which groups he should be held.[30]

Emerson, Day, and Wood had attempted to minimize racial and cultural tensions during the first three weeks of the fire policy by maintaining de facto segregation among the quarantine camps; to the extent possible, they unofficially put Chinese in one camp, Japanese in another, and Hawaiians in their own. As a practical matter, that also facilitated the job of the relief societies, who continued their practice of targeting their own. Only the white aid societies, which seemed especially solicitous of Hawaiian refugees, and the government itself, under the direction of the Board of Health, had been dispensing goods and services across racial and cultural lines. Emerson, Day, and Wood had sometimes also allowed individuals who were willing to pay for special services, including several whites and a few wealthy Chinese, to be quarantined separately in hotels commandeered for that purpose, rather than in the public camps. But the great fire forced the Board physicians to place people wherever space was available.[31]

At the Drill Shed camp, where approximately twelve hundred Japanese and Chinese refugees were situated, the Board received demands from the refugees themselves that the two groups be segregated. As a solution, the Board acquiesced in the construction of a high fence through the middle of the site. After that, the Drill Shed camp calmed considerably. Following separation, two of the Chinese residents in that camp wrote public letters assuring others in Honolulu that "all the Chinese [here] are very satisfied" and thanking the authorities—albeit somewhat sarcastically—for the "great kindness" of employing the Japanese to clean the camp every day while providing adequately for the Chinese. Visitors reported that the Kerosene Warehouse detention camp, which covered about four acres, resembled "a little cosmopolitan city." Since "segregation by nationalities has been the rule, . . . a tour of the place reminds one very much of a trip among the villages of different nationalities at the World's Fair." But this was a fair that no one had wanted to attend.[32]

12

The Triumvirate Struggles On

A s the state of emergency continued during the weeks following the
Chinatown fire and the constant problems of maintaining the quarantine camps began to mount, the medical triumvirate encountered distrust and uneasiness throughout Honolulu. Several whites started a rumor that dead bodies had been clandestinely spirited out of the Queen
Hotel, where a number of whites in quarantine were living under guard.
The three physicians issued formal public rebuttals and strong denials,
but the stories kept resurfacing in letters to the press. In private session,
Emerson, Day, and Wood seriously considered filing lawsuits against the
individuals who were accusing them of perpetrating a cover-up.[1]

The physicians' relations with recalcitrant whites declined further when
they learned from informers in executive session that some white women
who lived next to each other in a well-to-do neighborhood had been con-
spiring to ignore the emergency regulations regarding rats. The women
had been secretly burning dead and dying rats instead of reporting their
presence to the Citizens' Sanitary Commission or the Board of Health
and surrendering the carcasses for bacteriological examination. The women
did not want to risk the possibility that their homes might be condemned
as possible plague sites. When Ng Gee, a Chinese servant who worked for
one of them, died of plague, Emerson, Day, and Wood promptly invoked

his death as a reason to burn the women's houses. The women and their families were sent to quarantine camps.[2]

Accusations of fiscal irregularity and outright fraud on the part of some Citizens' Sanitary Commission agents peppered both the daily newspapers and the three physicians' daily meetings. Questions were raised about items allegedly being charged at public expense by sanitary agents in the field—including whiskey, cigars, and clothing—and about unequal rates of compensation for the small army of sanitary inspectors who continued to make their twice-daily rounds throughout the city. Even the most supportive businessmen in the city began to wonder aloud about the continued wisdom of spending vast sums of public money on nothing more than the say-so of three doctors, who lacked business acumen and faced no system of checks and balances. White opponents of the Dole administration pictured Hawaii on the brink of fiscal disaster as a consequence of the medical triumvirate's power to draw unlimited funds from the republic's treasury.[3]

More ominous still were rumors of petty blackmail, protection rackets, and shakedown schemes. Since nearly three-quarters of Honolulu's Asian residents had lived outside Chinatown all along, and more than half the Asian businesses in Honolulu were also located outside the quarantined zone, the lives and property of most of the city's Asians had not been directly affected by the great fire. Life for them continued more or less as usual, and the restrictions on them were not theoretically different from the continued restrictions on everyone else in Honolulu, including whites. Yet with Chinatown gone and plague cases continuing to break out around the city, Asians elsewhere in Honolulu grew understandably fearful of becoming targets themselves. A few Citizens' Sanitary Commission inspectors, or people posing as sanitary inspectors, took advantage of those fears by demanding gifts in exchange for omitting their businesses from the list of possible plague sites. One of these shakedown cases reached the front pages of the daily papers, where it touched off a round of mutual recrimination and interracial accusations. Since the Citizens' Sanitary Commission appointed exclusively male agents, rancor persisted as well over the propriety of their intimate personal inspections of women.[4]

Enduring divisions within the white medical establishment also hindered the ongoing campaign against plague. Although "the great doctors' meeting" three weeks earlier had produced a superficial impression of unity, serious philosophical disagreements persisted beneath the surface. On one side were those physicians who accepted both bacteriology and the Board's policy of selective burning. Those physicians typically volunteered to perform medical services under the Board's direction, often at considerable risk to themselves and with no compensation. On the other side were the physicians who continued to be skeptical of both bacteriology and the Board's approach to fighting plague. Many of the latter had absented themselves from "the great doctors' meeting," and even those who attended had shown themselves more interested in eliminating conditions they considered likely to enable disease than in trying to kill specific microbes, whose practical relevance they doubted.

These divisions complicated the handling of specific situations. R. E. Lockwood, for example, a frustrated subdistrict inspector who worked for the Citizens' Sanitary Commission, repeatedly reported a Chinese laundry and a Chinese store near the corner of Beretania and Emma streets to be unsanitary. He considered them "worse than in Chinatown a few weeks ago . . . foul," and wanted them burned. When the three physicians on the Board of Health failed to take action on his reports, Lockwood sought outside medical support to bolster his opinion, and readily received it from John McGrew, the former Medical Society president; Luis Alvarez, who back in December had written a public letter doubting Hoffman's bacteriological evidence of plague; and five other veteran physicians from the Medical Society. Despite pressure from Lockwood's seven allies, Emerson, Day, and Wood still refused to destroy the structures because no plague cases had occurred in them. Rather, they told the attorneys who represented the owners and tenants of the buildings to bring them up to code requirements or face penalties.[5]

Differences among Honolulu's white doctors surfaced again in an incident that occurred a week after the great fire. Late in the afternoon of January 27, arsonists ignited a largely abandoned block of shacks adjacent to a Chinese theater in the Aala district of the city. The resulting fire destroyed roughly thirty run-down structures over an area of about six acres before Chief Hunt's firefighters finally contained it with the help of employees from the Oahu Railroad Company, whose depot was downwind of the blaze. No one disputed that the ramshackle block ignited by the arsonist was an exceedingly foul site. Indeed, at the insistence of the Citizens' Sanitary Commission inspector for that part of the city, the Board's three physicians had previously designated the block as officially unsanitary. "But," as the *Advertiser* pointed out, "there had been no case of plague in [that block] and it had not been condemned to be burned." Instead, the Board physicians had tentatively planned to fill the area's cesspools, empty its garbage pits, and regrade the surrounding land, probably after the immediate crisis of the plague epidemic was over. In defiance of that decision, medical sanitationists sympathized publicly with the act of arson—which in their view accomplished something Emerson, Day, and Wood lacked enough guts to do.[6]

During the week following the Chinatown fire, when most businessmen and ordinary citizens were pitching in to help restabilize the city, the three exasperated and overtaxed doctors on the Board of Health "made emphatic reference to the lack of assistance on the part of the medical fraternity of Honolulu, that is, from the majority of those who are practicing physicians." The press tried to drum up support for the triumvirate running their city by pointing out that "important communications, delegations from Chinese and Japanese sources, reports of special committees and the detention camp superintendents, the issuance of instructions and orders, visiting different posts, listening to complaints and personally attending emergency calls for a physician, prove a burden which should be relieved as much as possible by others." But beyond those doctors who had been helping from the outset, no one came forward.[7]

The limited number of medical volunteers forced the Board's physicians to reduce the other services they usually provided the people of Honolulu. Prior to the plague crisis, for example, Henry Sloggett, a graduate of Edinburgh Medical School, had maintained the Board's Eye and Ear Infirmary. That infirmary treated indigent patients free of charge, primarily because Sloggett himself took no salary for his public services. But with so few medical professionals coming forward to help, the triumvirate needed Sloggett's assistance more urgently in the campaign against *pestis* than at the clinic—especially since Sloggett knew how to prepare bacteriological slides. So they were forced to close the infirmary and redeploy him in support of Hoffman. By the end of January, the triumvirate was so shorthanded that the stalwart band of volunteers who had stood with them since December began taking turns sleeping in the Board of Health office so someone would be on duty for plague-related emergencies at all times.[8]

Emerson, Day, and Wood bitterly resented the lack of cooperation—even outright opposition—they were receiving from so many of their European and American medical colleagues. Besieged on several fronts and facing enormous tasks ahead, their own morale flagged badly in the wake of the great fire. Since becoming Board president, Wood had been forced to abandon his private practice completely and was working essentially around the clock as Hawaii's de facto chief executive. Ever strong-willed and determined, he took challenges to the Board's policies personally, and his interviews with reporters grew noticeably testy as the city's press corps probed alleged mismanagement and questioned the medical triumvirate's decisions.

Emerson and Day also spent most of their waking hours on Board matters. The situation strained the family lives of all three doctors, exacting heavy financial and psychological sacrifices. Back on January 4, Emerson had written confidently to his sister about the campaign he and his two colleagues on the Board were waging against the plague epidemic. "I am not enough of a prophet to foresee when the end will be," he wrote. "But there *will* be an end, and we shall all see it and rejoice." Now, twenty days later, he was feeling considerably more despondent. Instead of reaffirmations of victory ahead, he wrote a last will and testament into his small notebook, declaring his wife Sarah his sole heir. He had Day solemnly witness the document.[9]

The relentless pressure of the plague campaign also took a heavy toll on the personal life of the Board's most crucial outside medical supporter, Carmichael from the Marine Hospital Service. With the city's crisis commanding more and more of his attention, his marriage of six months began to fall apart. What seemed like a marvelous match the previous July turned into a nightmare after the great fire, as the new Mrs. Carmichael exercised her violent temper in fits of outrage, sometimes storming off to stay with friends and threatening to divorce the public health doctor who seemed to be neglecting her.[10]

Though the situation in Honolulu following the great fire nearly overwhelmed the exhausted medical team battling *pestis*, the conflagration did retard the progress of the epidemic. The daily death tolls, which had been rising prior to January 20, abruptly leveled off and then declined through the end of the month. The day after the fire, an eight-month-old Chinese baby died of plague in his parents' home near the Oahu Railway station, but the three physicians decided the case had been introduced from Chinatown prior to the fire. They all knew the case personally, since the baby's father was one of their employees. For the entire week preceding the fire, he had been handling goods removed from condemned properties for fumigation and storage, so the doctors assumed that he had somehow tragically brought the disease home to his child. But to prevent the bacteria from establishing another new beachhead, the physicians felt they had no choice but to burn the family's house and quarantine the grieving parents.

To the great relief of Emerson, Day, and Wood, the resettlement camps remained free from fresh outbreaks of plague. Only one death from disease of any kind was reported in any of the city's sprawling camps: a twenty-three-year-old Japanese man who had lived in the same block as

Kaumakapili Church was found dead at the Kalihi camp the day after the fire, but whatever killed him was not plague. Emerson credited the lack of plague cases to the Board's insistence on thoroughly disinfecting both people and goods inside the camps, and to the policy of separating those who had direct contact with prior plague cases, such as "husbands & wives, sweethearts, and nurses," from those who did not.[11]

Elsewhere around the city, the epidemic slowed to sporadic cases, like that of Ng Gee, which popped up unpredictably in seemingly random places. Wherever they occurred, the three physicians continued to condemn the affected property and the fire department continued to burn what the Board condemned. On January 30, for example, firemen burned a shack above Wyllie Street where a Chinese man named Quong Fat Man had been found dead from plague. But that case worried the Board's physicians more than most because it seemed to suggest that some Chinese had resumed the practice of transporting plague patients away from residential or business properties, lest those properties be condemned. Their suspicions rose when passersby began to discover other Chinese bodies in improbable locations.[12]

The total number of deaths continued to dwindle through January, and by the end of the month both the English-language press and the Board's physicians were beginning to sound more optimistic than either had been since the great fire. On January 30, the front-page story of the *Advertiser* happily announced, "No Deaths Yesterday: Plague Seems to Be Abating." Daily editorials began looking to the future rather than commenting on the troubles of the previous day. Welcome news arrived from Washington, D.C., that the United States government would help underwrite any expenses incurred as a result of fighting the plague in its recently annexed archipelago. Citywide discussions also got underway about various long-term redevelopment ideas for the area destroyed in the great fire. Emerson, Day, and Wood held public meetings with Chinatown property owners to hear their opinions about redevelopment and listened for hours as engineers debated alternative plans for rebuilding the area with filtered water systems and sanitary sewers.[13]

The triumvirate's renewed optimism suffused a long private letter they wrote jointly on January 31 to their counterparts on the Board of Health of Sydney, Australia. Facing an attack of plague themselves, the Australians had written the Hawaiians for advice, which Emerson, Day, and Wood were now more than willing to offer. Their basic program for the last month, the Honolulu physicians told the Australians, "was to get the people out of their infested district and to provide for them in a Detention Camp in order to be able to disinfect such buildings as could be disinfected, and to destroy those that could not be rendered sanitary." The fact that plague had not broken out in the detention camps, deduced the Honolulu physicians, "seems to clearly show that it was the locality and not the people that were infected." Though we have lost twenty-six Chinese, seventeen Hawaiians, nine Japanese, one German, and one American, they wrote, our policies appear to have been effective, and "we now have the situation well in hand."[14]

Adding to hopes for the future were Walter Hoffman's ongoing experiments to develop a serum or an antidote for plague, using the samples of *pestis* bacteria he had been carefully collecting and cultivating as he performed his autopsies on the city's dead. Hoffman was working on variations of a process the British had tried to use in India in 1899, which involved culturing substantial amounts of plague bacteria; killing them by subjecting them to high heat; extracting fluids from the dead bacteria; and injecting the fluids, which were called Haffkine's serum after the developer of the technique, into humans in varying concentrations and amounts. Though the serum had done nothing to help patients already infected with plague, the injections had shown some generally positive results in immunizing healthy recipients against subsequently contracting the disease.[15]

Hoffman was trying to prepare enough of the serum not only to inoculate people staying in Honolulu, but also to offer inoculation to anyone who might now wish to leave the city. Since Honolulu remained an official plague port in the eyes of the world, people headed elsewhere would need a certificate of immunity to disembark at their destination. He also offered his serum to anyone from Honolulu who wanted permission to travel elsewhere on the island of Oahu. Angus Smedley, a Mormon missionary, remembered arriving at Honolulu during this period. After being inspected by quarantine officers, he and his friends went directly "to the Board of Health office and received an injection in our arms of Haffkins [*sic*] Prophylactic for the prevension [*sic*] of Bubonic Plague. Our arms pained us some and brought on a fever, but we were soon over it. We all took the injection so we could go to the Church Headquarters at Laie."[16]

Bright and ambitious, Hoffman—along with scores of other pioneer bacteriologists working at the same time all around the globe—hoped that his efforts might somehow produce bacteriology's next big breakthrough: the conquest of the legendary black death. But even if his own experiments with new methods of serum-making proved futile or insufficient, the young medical scientist knew that he would soon be receiving bacteriological reinforcements in the form of plague serums from elsewhere.

Through his friend Carmichael, he had asked the Marine Hospital Services laboratory in Washington, D.C., to send anything they came up with that might help; and through his own European contacts, he had received assurance from the Pasteur Institute laboratories in Paris that they would do the same.[17]

The situation in Honolulu looked sufficiently hopeful by the first week of February that Hoffman, who had gone a week without having to perform a postmortem exam, took time off from his work on the serum to get married. He had met his bride, Katherine McNeill, shortly before the plague crisis began, when as a member of the Boston Lyric Opera Company she had come to Honolulu to sing. She fell in love with both the city and the young German aristocrat—though she was more than twelve years older than he—and when their engagement was announced after the epidemic struck, she was quoted as saying, "Even the plague can't drive me out." McNeill indirectly strengthened the Board's strong medical ties to Chicago, since she had lived there as a child, the daughter of a doctor. Fittingly, Hoffman's close professional friend Day, another ex-Chicagoan, served as best man at the wedding.[18]

While the Hoffmans honeymooned, the missionary press thanked God for the "rigid and vigorous sanitary measures so strenuously carried on by the Board of Health, and actively aided by the intelligent citizens of Honolulu. Segregation, disinfection, purgation by fire, and the thorough twice a day inspection of every dwelling, have produced marvellous [*sic*] results. There seems to be the strongest prospect that our city will soon be entirely delivered from the 'Black Death,' and cease to be dread to all around us." Public discussion among Honolulu's white elites continued to focus on hotly debated alternative proposals for redeveloping Chinatown. Public discussion among refugees in the detention camps and among their spokesmen outside the camps shifted from recriminations to reparations.[19]

The city's optimistic mood collapsed abruptly on February 3, when J. Weir Robertson, a white grocery store employee, came down with plague. A quiet man who had been in Honolulu for twenty years and was said never to go out at night, Robertson lived in a residential area off upper Nuuanu Street, immediately behind the home of the head sanitary inspector for his neighborhood. Earlier that week Robertson had proclaimed himself the winner of an informal rat-catching contest among the downtown grocers, and his casual handling of the dead rodents almost certainly produced his case of plague. But no one knew anything about the rat-catching contest when president Wood responded personally to an urgent message sent to the Board of Health office by Robertson's physician. Wood quickly concurred with Robertson's doctor that the case was almost certainly plague and ordered the patient removed to the city plague hospital. Robertson's fourteen-year-old daughter and the nurse who was attending him were both sent to the Kalihi detention camp. Honolulu awoke to front-page headlines: "White Man Stricken . . . on Nuuanu Street."[20]

The same day Robertson came down with plague, the first shipment of plague serum arrived from abroad. The Marine Hospital Service in Washington, D.C., had forwarded a hundred vials of an "anti-pestique" serum, which the Pasteur Institute hoped would be effective against active cases of plague, and a thousand vials of Haffkine-type prophylactic serum. The French bacteriologists who produced this batch of Haffkine serum warned their American colleagues that people might feel ill soon after being injected with it, but they thought it would probably begin providing some immunity after ten days. Officially the serums were all sent to Carmichael, but he immediately put them at the disposal of his friends on the Honolulu Board of Health. Though the anti-pestique preparation was completely untested—its makers had requested a full report regarding its effects—Wood and Carmichael agreed to permit Robertson's physician to administer the purported antidote to his patient. No one knew how much serum was supposed to be used under any given conditions, but the three physicians settled on two vials for Robertson—a bit less than a quarter of a cupful—which his doctor then injected into his back with a large hypodermic needle. As the press reported, with unintended understatement, "The medical fraternity will watch developments in Mr. Robertson's case with interest on account of the trial being given the new serum."[21]

Since the prompt administration of the prophylactic serums seemed less urgent than prompt administration of the anti-pestique that might save Robertson's life, the doctors decided to test the Haffkine preparation on a guinea pig before administering it to humans. Preparation of these prophylactic serums was still rather ad hoc, and batches were known to vary in strength and side effects, hence the warning that accompanied this batch. If the guinea pig survived, the Board's own physicians, starting with president Wood, offered themselves for the initial human trials. The three physicians also learned from the French consul in Honolulu that his government had instructed the Pasteur Institute in Paris to send twenty-five vials of a different batch of anti-pestique directly to the consul for use in Hawaii as he saw fit. Those doses were expected on the next steamer from

San Francisco, and the French consul would almost certainly offer them to the physicians on the Board of Health. Finally, Hoffman's own serum preparations were expected to be available shortly.[22]

Results from the Robertson experiment were not long in coming: he died within twenty-four hours of his two injections. A postmortem examination confirmed that his body was riddled with the aftereffects of plague. Perhaps, speculated the *Advertiser*, "the remedy lost some of its virtue in transit, just as vaccine matter is said to do." Truly fair tests would have to wait "until the fresh serum being prepared by Dr. Hoffman is available." Also ominous was a laboratory report that arrived on the day of Robertson's death regarding the recent demise of a Chinese man. Doctors at the time had not attributed Wong Chin's death to plague, since they had not found any plague bacteria in their initial examination of his remains. But as a safety precaution, they had dropped some of his bodily fluids into a "culture tube" for later exploration. The bacteria that subsequently developed in the culture tube proved to be unmistakably those associated with bubonic plague. Retroactively, Wong Chin was declared a plague victim.[23]

The day after Robertson died, the Board heard about three more fresh cases of possible plague. One was a Hawaiian man who had been at the Drill Shed camp for eleven days. The other two men were a recently arrived white American laborer and a Japanese worker. Since there was some doubt whether the Hawaiian case from the quarantine camp was actually plague (which it turned out not to be), the Board's physicians decided to try the anti-pestique on only the American and the Japanese, both of whom clearly had the disease. This time they administered just one vial of serum to each, in a single injection. Unfortunately, the results were the same as in Robertson's case.[24]

The American and the Japanese had both worked at the Pantheon Stables, one of the six largest stables operating in downtown Honolulu. Emerson, Day, and Wood were now reminded by their sanitary inspectors that Wong Chin had also worked there and that Quong Fat Man had frequently slept there. As a result, the three physicians overrode an earlier command that the Pantheon Stables be thoroughly disinfected as a precautionary measure and instead ordered them burned. This was a serious economic decision in a city that still ran entirely on horsepower. The Pantheon's remaining employees were sent under guard to quarantine camps.[25]

Later that day the triumvirate learned about Robertson's amateur rat-catching contests and surmised that rats might also be implicated in the

Pantheon deaths. Though they did not know what was going on, the three physicians figured they had nothing to lose and perhaps something to gain by stepping up their previously announced efforts to poison rats. They also cautioned the public to use shovels when disposing of dead rats in order to avoid touching them directly. In an effort to understand the mysterious relationship between rats and plague, Hoffman began meticulously cataloguing the exact locale of all dead rats reported to Board headquarters. But everyone was forced to admit that it had "been an unfortunate day in health department circles."[26]

As the pattern of sporadic deaths returned, so did tensions within the city. Charles J. Creighton, a local attorney representing Chinese residents accused of violating emergency health orders, launched a flamboyant public challenge of his own to the authority of Citizens' Sanitary Commission inspectors—and hence to the absolute powers of the Board of Health—by threatening to shoot anyone, including designated medical inspectors, who attempted to enter his home. Other anti-Dole whites joined in, accusing the three physicians on the Board of Health of losing control of the situation, and condemning the Citizens' Sanitary Commission as little more than a vigilante mob operating under the evil influence of Hawaii's own "Mr. Pain," Lorrin Thurston. The city's trolley company balked at the triumvirate's mandatory disinfection procedures, which kept downtown business at a standstill. Allegations of fiscal abuse resurfaced and were in turn counterchallenged by the Board's special Finance Committee. The latter refused, for example, to pay claims for the pick-helves that were given out by hardware merchants to passing citizens on the day of the great Chinatown fire, on the grounds that the Board would not have authorized such actions.[27]

Anxieties continued to rise during the first week of February, when people began to realize that the refugees from the great fire were nearing the end of their three-week quarantine period. While everyone was relieved that no additional cases of plague had broken out inside the camps—which, among other things, would have lengthened the period of quarantine—they also knew that the vast majority of the refugees soon to be released had no homes to return to and few resources of their own. Frightened members of the Dole administration floated the possibility of calling for additional U.S. troops or activating the Hawaiian national guard, in case the liberated refugees went on a rampage. But critics mocked the idea: "Is the government of the Republic of Hawaii prepared to admit that the Asiatic contingent which the magnificent labor system of the Republic has brought to this city is so large and evil minded that it cannot be controlled by local authorities?" Emerson, Day, and Wood let the proposal die.[28]

On February 8, the Board began releasing Chinatown fire refugees from detention camps. Evacuees were not forced out, but they were encouraged to leave if they could find alternative arrangements. With questions of reparations and public maintenance already looming large in private discussions among the Board's members and in debates between the Board's physicians and the Council of State, Emerson, Day, and Wood were reluctant to set the precedent of providing indefinitely for everyone who had sustained losses as a consequence of their antiplague policies. Even so, nearly 700 of the roughly 1,850 refugees released from the Kalihi camp returned immediately, and the triumvirate agreed to continue supporting them.[29]

Fortunately, the initial exodus from the camps went smoothly. Far from rampaging, some of the Chinese refugees presented gifts of appreciation to their former guards as they left the camps. The *Tan Shang Xi Bao Long Ji* [Hawaiian Chinese News] admonished refugees not to defy the Board of Health by trying to return to their former homes, and the Board's physicians cooperated actively with the Chinese Aid Society to provide transitional support for those who chose to leave the camps. Consul Yang and Vice-Consul Gu administered a substantial fund that provided essentials to Chinese evacuees, though Yang was later accused of diverting large amounts to his own coffers.[30]

Japanese consul Saito Miki provided cash payments to departing Japanese refugees, so they in turn might compensate countrymen who took them in. He also began seeking work for Japanese around the city or, failing that, on plantations elsewhere in the archipelago. Chinese, Japanese, and Hawaiian relief societies again came forward to help provide assistance for their respective constituencies. Employment bureaus opened in the camps and managed to find jobs for 120 of the first 440 refugees released from quarantine; newspapers thereafter regularly published lists of available workers and their principal skills.[31]

Most of the released evacuees had to make do as best they could, and many had no friend or relative to take them in. The editor of *Ke Aloha Aina* wept at the "pathetic condition" of some of the people released from quarantine. They walked the streets aimlessly during the day and slept outdoors "under kiawe trees and on akulikuli grass" at night, victims, in his opinion, of the "cruelty of this annexationist government that some Hawaiians boast is a good government." He was especially saddened that Hawaiian refugees were being treated callously by "hard-hearted Hawaiians" serving in the Dole government's police force. With no home to go back to, some of the Hawaiian refugees from Chinatown would still be living in the Kalihi barracks two years later and trying to persuade the government to let them homestead there permanently.[32]

A reporter for the *Independent* met a Japanese refugee "who looked pale and miserable and scantily dressed." The reporter was disconcerted, "because a month ago we knew him as a thrifty citizen, always in good employ, and always neatly dressed." The Japanese man told the reporter "that he had just been released from the detention camp, to find his house in Chinatown burned down, his furniture and clothing gone up in smoke with the money which altogether represented the savings of seventeen years of faithful labor in these islands." With tears in his eyes, the man "pointed towards the bleak desert between Nuuanu street and the River street and said, 'I have lost my home, my property, and even my job.'"[33]

Through all of this, Emerson, Day, and Wood stoutly maintained twice-daily inspections of the entire city and declined to restore full business hours. Schools remained closed and transit facilities sharply curtailed. Wherever and whenever Board-appointed physicians confirmed new plague cases, the triumvirate continued its policy of relocating any surviving residents to quarantine camps and burning the site. As people continued to die, the dispirited press was reduced to writing about how well the city's human crematorium had been functioning during the crisis. Built in just four days back in December, the facility was praised by a weary Wood, who took sardonic pride in pointing out that Honolulu's crematorium was superior even to the one in Tokyo, Japan—hardly the sort of boast he had been hoping to make.[34]

Among the few bright spots for the white elites in Honolulu was the recovery of Armstrong Smith, a popular young man barely out of school. At considerable risk to himself, Smith had volunteered to run the Board's special plague, or so-called pest, hospital since its creation back in December. He had been continuously at that post ever since. When he suddenly took sick during the second week of February, people feared the worst. But Smith recovered, and the grateful Americans of the city took up a collection to send the young man to medical school once the plague emergency was over.[35]

Discouraged by the enormity of the problems ahead, everyone in Honolulu realized that the plague-induced state of emergency was far from over. Watching the city stagger on, the Roman Catholic bishop of Hawaii wrote sadly to friends in England about "the black death" in the Pacific.

"For more than a month we have been exposed to the ravages of this fearful visitation; God alone knows when we shall get rid of it," he reported. "Meanwhile the government and its Board of Health are making desperate efforts to stamp out the disease; they do not hesitate to set on fire all the infected quarters, and if they go on burning down at this rate, one half of the city will soon have disappeared. Up till a few days ago, the victims were Chinese and Japanese or Kanakas [Hawaiians], but now several white people have been attacked," and the population was clearly on edge. "Poor people!" he concluded, "they put more trust in their science than in the mercy of God."[36]

13

The Frustrations of Mopping Up

A s if the frustrations they faced in Honolulu were not enough, Emerson, Day, and Wood continued to receive occasional rumors of plague elsewhere in the archipelago. But beyond asserting their authority—as they did on Hawaii—and insisting on strict quarantine procedures, the doctors had not directly intervened in the daily affairs of the outer islands, where most residents still wanted nothing to do with Honolulu in any event until the epidemic was over. But by early February reports from the island of Maui had become too serious to ignore, so Wood himself decided to make an unannounced trip to Kahului, the island's principal city, on February 11. He took along Charles Louis Garvin, who had been one of the first physicians in private practice to volunteer his services to the Board back in December.[1]

When Wood and Garvin arrived in Kahului, they learned that six people had died during the preceding week, all apparently from plague. Four victims were Chinese, the other two were Japanese; all six had lived in Kahului's small Chinatown district. Wood examined another gravely ill Chinese patient in that district, who died three hours later. The doctors then performed postmortem examinations on three of the victims and— to confirm their diagnosis—viewed "slides made by Dr. Garvin [which] showed the bacilli of plague in large numbers." All of the bodies were then immediately cremated upon a pyre of railroad ties.

Acting formally as president of the Board of Health, and invoking the emergency powers the Board possessed throughout Hawaii, Wood called an impromptu meeting of the local physicians in town, the local version of the Citizens' Sanitary Association, the sheriff of Maui, and "all the white population that could be spared from patrolling" Kahului's own hastily established quarantine zone. Together they resolved that Kahului's Chinatown, an area of about three acres, could not be effectively disinfected, so Wood concluded that the "only treatment" available was "disposal of the place by fire." An ad hoc appraising committee removed "such papers and valuables as . . . can safely be disinfected," then estimated the worth of the district's buildings and any unsalvageeable merchandise they contained. A. N. Kapoikai, who had formerly served in the old Hawaiian senate, took charge of preparing quarantine camps for the people about to be displaced.

The assessors completed their task in less than an hour, and Kahului's Chinatown was ignited. A San Francisco attorney who happened to be visiting Kahului at the time was surprised to see "far less objections made to the removal and far less resistance" on the part of the Chinatown residents than he had expected. The decision affected roughly two hundred residents, mostly Chinese and Japanese, along with a few Hawaiians and one white, all of whom were relocated to "comfortable" quarantine quarters on the grounds of the town's horse racing track. The sheriff was instructed to find anyone who had left the Chinatown district for other parts of the island during the previous week, round them up, and add them to the residents being quarantined. Wood then formally deputized six local physicians and twelve civilians "as agents of the Board of Health" before returning to Honolulu the following day. Wood left Garvin behind, "with a complete outfit of all that is needed for microscopical and postmortem work," to command the battle against plague on Maui.[2]

Returning to Honolulu, Wood found the situation improving. Refugees were continuing to leave the detention camps without incident. With fewer people to detain under quarantine and no widespread civil unrest breaking out, the three physicians reduced the number of national guardsmen they had called to active duty. On February 15, they opened several streets that had been closed to the public since the Chinatown fire. By February 19, Honolulu had gone twelve days without a death, so the triumvirate ordered the Citizens' Sanitary Commission to cut their citywide inspections to once a day. But Wood and his colleagues remained cautious. Over the objection of educators, for example, the physicians insisted that Honolulu's schools stay closed, and they continued to direct spot fires at sites linked to earlier outbreaks.[3]

With the epidemic apparently receding, Emerson, Day, and Wood spent increasing amounts of their time embroiled in financial issues and haggling over future developments. The city's shippers, for example, began to badger the Board to loosen import regulations and asserted that they would self-police the city's wharves and warehouses in exchange for the resumption of unhindered trade. Exasperated by such bullying, Wood rebuked the shippers publicly. "I believe that the steamship companies and the merchants of Honolulu . . . are inclined to ship as much freight as they can and escape the restrictions if possible," he told newspaper reporters summoned to the Board's office. "I don't think they are acting in the manner citizens or companies should, who wish to have the plague suppressed soon." Privately to his two colleagues at their daily meeting, Wood put the problem more succinctly: "The merchants [are] getting restless." The physicians also had to spend time dealing with reports of price gouging on the part of retailers and investigating allegations that some physicians in the city were charging Asian patients for services they were supposed to be providing for free.[4]

Dwarfing all other economic issues, however, were the various redevelopment plans for Chinatown, the Board's previous commitment to improving the city's hygienic infrastructure, and the desire on all sides to solve the thorny problem of reparations stemming from all of the Board-ordered fires. On February 19, the three physicians took a major step toward the future by earmarking still another $500,000 for sewer construction in the Chinatown area, plus an additional $100,000 for plague-related expenses. In a republic whose national treasury held only about $3 million to begin with, the magnitude of the sums encumbered during the plague emergency indicated just how completely and how boldly the three medical men had taken control of Hawaii.[5]

On the same day the three physicians committed "the existing government" to costly projects that would continue after the epidemic ended, three of their volunteer physicians in the field almost simultaneously reported three more deaths from plague. After nearly two weeks without any fatalities, those reports were a discouraging setback, particularly because the body of one of the victims, a man named Ah Hung, had been found at the Hawaiian Hotel Stables. Those stables housed over eighty horses and served most of the city's tourists, as well as many of the city's downtown businesses. If burned, they would be a highly visible symbol to outsiders of how serious the city's plague problem still remained, so the three physicians did not want to condemn them without strong evidence of plague. The other Asian employees at the Hotel Stables claimed that Ah Hung once worked there, but had not been seen for weeks prior to his death, and hence could not have contracted plague there. Company pay records substantiated their claims.

To resolve the issue, the triumvirate staged a formal hearing, listened to witnesses, and took statements regarding the status of the Hotel Stables. While the evidence about Ah Hung's whereabouts and death remained inconclusive, the hearing brought to light the fact that a prior plague death had occurred there in January. Fearing for their jobs, Japanese employees had concealed that death and secretly substituted one of their friends for the man who died. The doppelgänger answered to the name of the dead plague victim, and the local white sanitary inspector never discovered the ruse. Emerson, Day, and Wood disagreed over what to do. President Wood was prepared "to strain a point" in order to do away with these or any stables "in the heart of the city," where he thought they did not belong anyway. The more cautious Emerson felt they lacked sufficient evidence to burn the stables immediately. As a compromise, they agreed on Day's proposal for a tight quarantine around the stables, coupled with a wait-and-see policy.

The decision to delay condemnation of the Hotel Stables touched off another embarrassingly public showdown between the sanitationist attitudes of the vast majority of whites and the Board physicians' more bacteriologically discriminating policy. McGrew, the Board's old medical nemesis, publicly accused Emerson, Day, and Wood of dangerous inconsistency. "It is well known that two persons who afterwards died of the plague had been on the premises for a longer or shorter time," he stated. "Burn them by all means." W. E. Taylor, another of the traditional physicians who had kept his distance from the Board, took a similar position. "I suppose the Board has some good reason for not destroying the Hotel stables," he commented to a newspaper interviewer, "but I haven't any idea what that reason is. . . . For my part, I most emphatically say, burn the stables."[6]

The Citizens' Sanitary Commission drafted a formal letter of protest against what they regarded as an unwarranted departure from "the radical policy heretofore inaugurated . . . in destroying premises found, upon reasonable evidence, after investigation, to be infected by plague." In an ugly session full of angry demands and sarcastic replies, Thurston clashed openly with Emerson and Day. In the eyes of some, Thurston appeared bent upon using the Hotel Stables incident to put his Citizens' Sanitary Commission in command of the city in place of the Board of Health that created and authorized it. For five days, editorial after editorial implored the triumvirate to accept the demands of the Citizens' Sanitary Commission and burn the Hawaiian Hotel Stables, as they had previously burned the Pantheon Stables. As the rancor grew, U.S. military observers tersely notified Washington: "Situation at Honolulu horrible."[7]

While the pro-government press pounded the doctors with headlines like "Duty Calls For Fire," another Chinese employee of the Hotel Stables came down with plague. This man, Ah Sing, died on February 26, and the Board held a special meeting to reconsider its wait-and-see position. Testimony was again confused and contradictory. Clearly, some parties were not telling the truth about which workers lived or did not live at the Hotel Stables; others challenged the identification of the dead man. A thoroughly exasperated Wood finally decided to accept the word of Ah Sop, a witness whom Wood knew personally, and concluded on the basis of Ah Sop's statements that the Hotel Stables should indeed be confirmed as a plague site. Though influential lawyers for the Hawaiian Hotel argued fiercely in favor of alternative forms of disinfection, the three physicians voted to burn the stable, a decision hailed in the press as overdue, and correct.[8]

Deaths from plague continued to occur from the end of February into the early weeks of March, though they did so in diminishing numbers and without apparent patterns. The seemingly random location of the deaths raised once again the possibility that Honolulu's remaining plague bacteria were being conveyed around the city in Asian foodstuffs, something the Board president had suspected all along. In his report about the situation on Maui, Wood had pointedly mentioned that the people of Kahului felt certain that plague entered their community on a shipment of Asian fruits and vegetables that had arrived shortly before the initial outbreaks. But the other two physicians tabled a resolution that would have committed them formally to the "official opinion" that "the continued cropping [up] of cases of plague in Honolulu seems logically chargeable to the presence of infection in Asiatic food stuffs." Moreover, despite Wood's protestations, his colleagues again declined to endorse the destruction of all "such Oriental food products as lie under strong suspicion of contamination." Deployment of two new disinfecting devices for foods and merchandise at wharves and warehouses, one a hot-air compartment and the other a steam-pressure chamber, helped mollify the Board president.[9]

With renewed deaths came renewed burning. On February 26, a Chinese man named Kee Mong was found dead of plague in a tenement house. The patient had been seen once prior to his death by the ever-needling McGrew, who claimed he declined "a large fee" offered by the dead man's friends "if he would give a death certificate that the patient died of some other disease." The Board physicians ordered the fire department to burn the tenement where Kee Mong was found, as well as the buildings on the Wong Kwai rice plantation, where the dead man had stayed while he was sick. The other residents of the tenement and the employees at the rice plantation were detained in quarantine camps. When a worker at the New England Bakery came down with plague, that shop was burned, as was the Globe Stables, where physicians discovered yet another case of plague. Employees of both businesses were sent to quarantine camps.[10]

As the epidemic continued into March, the Board's physicians grew fearful that *pestis* might be riding dust particles around the city. To prevent that possibility, they ordered contractors to sprinkle the city's streets at night with a 5-percent solution of sulfuric acid. After the first few nights a local professor, who otherwise admired the Board physicians' commitment to the latest science, pointed out that Hawaii's porous and nonacidic soils would quickly neutralize the acid. Chagrined, the three physicians accepted his substitute measure: the application of unslacked lime at ten tons to the acre. If plague bacteria that had escaped the fires were lurking in the soil, the lime might kill them. Critics accused the Board's physicians of still not knowing how the epidemic was continuing to spread— having gone after buildings, rats, food, people, personal items, and now dust. They were right. But the critics had no answers either.[11]

Through these continuing frustrations, Emerson, Day, and Wood clung to hopes that laboratory scientists would develop effective serums and antidotes to counteract their invisible enemy. On March 5, eight doctors associated with the Board of Health, including Hoffman, met at Sloggett's house to organize the new Honolulu Microscopical Society.[12] The society's statement of purpose amounted to a manifesto on behalf of bacteriology-based medicine.

> The time has come when all progressive physicians, surgeons, general practitioners and specialists alike, must [have access to] skill in microscopic technique. . . . In no other way can they conscientiously perform their duty to those whose lives are placed in their hands, and fully meet the reasonable requirements of advancing medical science. . . . [W]ithout [microscopy] the practice of medicine and surgery would be little better than guess work. The microscope has wrought a complete transformation in the once dominant ideas concerning the treatment of epidemic and contagious diseases and especially may we boast of the truly wonderful advances made in bacteriology.[13]

Members of the Microscopical Society hoped to join Hoffman's efforts to find antidotes to plague. They knew that the U.S. Marine Hospital Service was trying to perfect something known as Yersin's serum—after the co-discoverer of *pestis*—which involved injecting horses with plague and extracting blood fluids that the horses produced to resist the bacteria. A similar technique had proved successful in creating anti-diphtheria serums. Since it would be several months before any of the new horse-based serum could reach Hawaii, the Microscopical Society decided to conduct experiments of their own in Honolulu. In the meantime, they waited for the next shipment of Haffkine's preventive serum that U.S. surgeon general Walter Wyman had promised more than a month ago.[14]

On March 12, the new batch, containing almost two thousand doses, finally arrived by ship from San Francisco. Since the first serums had produced such discouraging outcomes, Honolulu residents had grown skeptical of antiplague inoculations. Indeed, the *Evening Bulletin* revealed that Garvin found live *pestis* in the earlier batch of Haffkine's serum, though Garvin suggested somewhat unconvincingly that his slides might have been contaminated by a plague autopsy he had conducted shortly before preparing them. To win the public back, the three physicians decided to stage a dramatic demonstration.[15]

The day after the serum arrived, Wood summoned the press corps and announced that he would take the first injection from the new batch. He "thought it was only fair that he should be the first man to undergo the treatment and in this manner demonstrate to the public that the serum was harmless and unobjectionable, and at the same time ascertain in the interests of science and an inquiring populace just what the effect of taking the prophylactic would be." Day, Wood's lifelong friend, medical partner, and colleague on the Board of Health, accompanied the president into the Board's bacteriological laboratory and self-consciously declared that "as a worshipper of science, . . . [he] was not going to be left behind by his fellow-practitioner." The two doctors then agreed to inject each other, leaving their senior colleague in charge. "Professionally the two doctors were not in the least afraid," commented a reporter who witnessed the scene, but he detected "under their physicians' nonchalance . . . just the smallest amount of trepidation."[16]

Because public demonstration was the purpose of the episode, the press tracked the progress of the two physicians closely. Both men became seriously ill. Wood fought a high fever and extreme lethargy long enough to put in a symbolic appearance at Board headquarters, despite feeling "as if he had swallowed all the bacilli in the dictionary." He lacked the stamina to stay very long, and his obvious discomfort and visible shaking combined to produce exactly the headline he did not want: "Dr. Wood Sick." The press surmised that Wood's severe reaction to the serum probably resulted from his "arduous labor" and "tremendous responsibility" over the last three months, a period during which "Dr. Wood [has been] doing just about as much as it is possible for a man to do, in fact the doctor has been overworking himself." The press reported that "the people at large" were inquiring earnestly about Wood and "manifest[ed] a deep interest in his experiment with the serum." Day was a bit less violently ill, but remained in seclusion, telling reporters he was "uncomfortable."[17]

Following two more days of intense discomfort, Wood finally phoned the *Advertiser* to say he was recovering. Editorials expressed relief that "the head of the fighters against the plague" would shortly be back on the job. The following week, with less publicity, Hoffman also injected himself with serum; he also got quite sick, but recovered fully. Relieved and reassured, ordinary citizens began cautiously to come forward to receive inoculations, which Board physicians provided at no cost.[18]

Most numerous among the early volunteers for inoculation were Honolulu's Japanese residents. Since the Board made inoculation a condition of travel to the outlying islands of the archipelago, the English-language press surmised that the possibility of obtaining jobs on the plantations of Kauai, Maui, and Hawaii must have been motivating the Japanese. While those assumptions were partly correct, whites beyond the Board of Health seemed completely unaware that cultural factors among the Japanese themselves were also playing a significant role. Well before the arrival of plague, Japanese physicians in the city had regularly filled *Yamato Shimbun*, the leading Japanese-language newspaper, with advertisements touting their use of the latest and most scientific medical technologies, including bacteriological inoculations.[19]

Mori Iga was a good example. Mori had attended the Japanese Naval Medical School in the late 1880s, where the Meiji government insisted on teaching the latest Western curriculum. He then earned his MD in 1891 at Cooper Medical School in San Francisco before coming to Hawaii to serve as a government physician for the surge of incoming Japanese laborers. Mori had also gone briefly to London in 1898 to study at University Hospital. For several years prior to the arrival of plague, Mori had publicly advertised himself in Honolulu as a particular specialist in vaccinations and inoculations. When plague did appear, *Yamato Shimbun* reported the efforts underway in bacteriological laboratories worldwide to develop vaccines to combat the disease. Kitasato's heroic stature as a scientific warrior battling the pandemic back home with bacteriological weapons also helped make Honolulu's Japanese colony (as they called themselves) more accepting of bacteriology, and hence of serum inoculations, than any other group in the city.[20]

As more and more people underwent the prophylactic inoculation without grave side effects, the initial lines of ten volunteers a day turned into scores. Anonymous individuals floated the idea of making inoculations universal and compulsory, but their suggestions were dropped when opposition to mandatory inoculation surfaced almost immediately in the English-language press. Even so, the Board physicians were running out of serum by the end of March. They sent an urgent message to the Hawaiian consul in San Francisco to try to obtain another 250 flasks from Washington. If that was impossible, the consul was instructed to cable the Pasteur Institute in Paris with the same request. In the meantime, Carmichael agreed to augment the city's supply of serum from his own military stores. By the end of April, the Board had inoculated close to two thousand people in Honolulu and was considering charging future patients for the service to generate revenue for the financially strained government.[21]

In contrast to the preventive serum, the therapeutic applications proved ineffective against cases of plague already contracted. When Herman Levy, a day clerk at the Hawaiian Hotel, came down with what initially appeared to be plague, he asked to be admitted to the special pest hospital for treatment. Hoffman administered several doses of a new serum he hoped to use against active cases of plague, and Levy improved. Emerson, Day, and Wood rejoiced that the sharp young bacteriologist, whom they trusted even before the plague arrived, had now found something that might help stop the epidemic. But when Levy made a rapid recovery with no further evidence of plague, even Hoffman concluded that Levy had probably been sick with something else all along, so the serum had not cured him of plague.[22]

Egged on by McGrew, who later examined Levy and declared him to be suffering from pneumonia, Levy's father, a prominent rabbi in San Francisco, subsequently protested the triumvirate's treatment of his son, alleging poor diagnosis, discrimination, and—most aggressively—the administration of dangerous inoculations. Herman Levy himself, however, defended the Board's physicians completely, pointing out that he had received the best possible care and attention, and he offered the firm opinion that Hoffman had done the right thing to administer his serum under the circumstances. Yet Levy's case could not be counted as a triumph for the plague antidote. While Board physicians continued to administer various batches of serum to other plague patients, none of the injections retarded cases already contracted.[23]

Following the widespread administration of preventive inoculations, the number of new plague cases resumed its downward trend. The three physicians did not know whether the reduction resulted from the cumulative effects of their ongoing fire policy, from the inoculations, or from a combination of both, but they were grateful for a chance to relax some of their emergency measures and prepare the city for an eventual return to normal routines. To a large extent, their official actions merely ratified what was taking place anyway as the epidemic slowed. Outside Honolulu, residents stopped enforcing quarantines that were theoretically still in effect. Inside the city, daily health reports began to fall off as Citizens' Sanitary Commission inspectors felt less urgency to keep repeating "no new cases."[24]

Emerson, Day, and Wood happily took the declining number of inspectors' reports as a reason to disband the troublesome Citizens' Sanitary Commission altogether and replace their legions of volunteer inspectors with a small corps of paid agents—including some women (the Citizens' Sanitary Commission had refused to appoint female inspectors)—whom they could choose personally and monitor directly. Since the number of permanent paid agents would be no more than a small fraction of the number of volunteer inspectors that previously circulated through the city under the aegis of the Citizens' Sanitary Commission, this decision effectively ended the city's state of constant surveillance. In lieu of continuous oversight, the three physicians announced a reward of a hundred dollars for anyone reporting a suspected plague case. "Such an offer," they reasoned among themselves in private session, "may induce a man's friends or enemies to report his case."[25]

The three physicians also permitted contractors to resume construction in most parts of the city—though not yet in Chinatown—provided all structures met their tough new sanitary regulations. The city's newspapers printed those revised codes in serial form throughout the month. Included in the first round of new building permits were several that went to Chinese and Japanese citizens. Even at the end of the month, however, despite intense pressure and another exchange of "strong talk" with Honolulu's shippers, the Board physicians refused to loosen their tight restrictions on trade, citing the continued outbreak of occasional plague cases. Indeed, the very day the merchants had their most acrimonious showdown with the triumvirate so far, two new cases of plague appeared. Both patients died the following day, March 25.[26]

The Frustrations of Mopping Up

Near the end of March, Wood announced his intention to resign as president of the Board of Health. He was depleted, he said, physically and financially. He had expected the battle against plague to last about a month, but it had lasted more than three months. He had been forced to abandon his own medical practice, and he seldom had any time to spend with his wife and two small children. Having led the most intense part of the campaign against plague and having served as de facto dictator of Hawaii through some of the most trying months of its history, he was exhausted. "I would not serve again for $10,000," he told the press, and asked his two compatriots on the Board to find someone else to oversee the remaining mop-up operations.

Editorials praised Wood and called for "some substantial recognition" of this physician who "battled the plague at its worst . . . without salary." His colleagues appointed Wood to a special committee to nominate a new president, thereby insuring him a major voice in the selection of his successor. The pro-government press speculated wishfully that longtime Dole confidante George W. Smith would probably take over, but instead Wood secured the appointment of his lieutenant from the Kahului episode, thirty-one-year-old Charles Garvin, to serve as a sort of executive secretary or ex officio president. Garvin was recalled from Maui to relieve his mentor from the management of day-to-day affairs, allowing Emerson and Day to ceremoniously decline Wood's formal resignation as their official president.[27]

Garvin's elevation as de facto president kept a bacteriologically oriented medical doctor at the helm of Hawaii's ruling authority, but the major trials he faced through the rest of March and April turned out to be financial and legal rather than explicitly medical. From the outset of the plague crisis, and certainly since the initial implementation of the fire policy, Emerson, Day, and Wood had operated under the assumption that losses imposed by governmental agencies for purposes of protecting the general welfare would be compensated. Assessors had regularly and formally recorded the value of all condemned property prior to its destruction, and that practice was continued for the duration of the emergency. But in addition to predictable disputes over who owned what and exactly how much it was worth, the Board's physicians faced two much larger and more difficult problems: Where was the money for reparations to come from? And how should they determine the value of losses not assessed in advance, which included everything lost in the Chinatown fire?

Claims for lost property resulting from the great fire strained the capacity of the file cabinets at Board headquarters. Many of the largest losses were claimed by white landowners, whose rented buildings in the quarantined district had been destroyed completely. Another source of claims came from business owners, white and Asian, whose stores, merchandise, or production facilities had been in Chinatown, though they themselves lived elsewhere. The largest and most desperate group of claimants, however, were the refugees themselves, most of whom began submitting claims while still interned in the quarantine camps. During earlier controlled fires, the Chinese and Japanese consulates had worked out a way for their constituents to submit their own property inventories, which then functioned as a check against official appraisals made by Board-appointed assessors. Both consuls now invited similar constituent-drafted tallies of all losses from the great fire.

The efforts of Yang Wei Pin and Saito Miki rapidly amassed bulging folders full of fire claims, which they regularly delivered to the Board's office. Many of the claims were extremely detailed, listing such specific items as straw sandals and socks valued at ten cents. But the three physicians had no way of verifying the self-generated claims, which was a problem, since all parties—including the Chinese and Japanese press—realized that many of them were almost certainly inflated. Unable to solve that problem in the short run, the medical triumvirate simply accepted the mounting volume of claims without comment. They still had the plague itself to deal with, and they were perfectly willing to let other agencies adjudicate reparations sometime in the future.[28]

Also behind the decision to defer claims was a pronouncement from the leading American insurance companies doing business in Hawaii. When they learned what was happening in Honolulu, key representatives of those firms met in San Francisco and collectively agreed to reject all claims lodged by policyholders as the result of Board-ordered fires. The insurance companies took the position that public authorities had purposely ignited the fires and would therefore have to pay for any damages the fires had done, intentional or accidental. Some of the city's policyholders still held hopes that insurance companies based in Europe and Asia might be more generous, but the news was a heavy blow to Honolulu's American elites, who knew that their own treasury was down to almost nothing as a result of actions taken by Emerson, Day, and Wood during the last three months.[29]

Stonewalled by the insurance industry, some of the fire victims took their damage claims instead to the Hawaiian Republic's supreme court, even though the status of that court was unclear in the congressional resolution of annexation. Ducking the issue, the Hawaiian justices ruled on March 31 that nothing should be done until President McKinley decided whether or not to commit federal funds to help the annexed archipelago deal with its fire reparations. Since McKinley was actively engaged in the ongoing efforts of Hawaii's "existing government" to secure formal territorial status under the American Constitution, the supreme court justices had reason to hope Washington might bail them out if they played for time.

To mollify those who wanted to see some preliminary action at the local level, however, Dole himself took a position different from that of the supreme court. Early in April, he announced the creation of a special ad hoc court of claims to begin processing requests for compensation for losses incurred in Board-ordered fires. Though many claimants wanted prompt action, or at least some short-term assistance to help them rebuild their lives, Dole's promulgation of a special court met stiff resistance from the outset. Attorneys for English-speaking claimants protested the legal status of the special court and squabbled over how justices should be appointed to it. When the white merchants and landlords realized that the special court did not intend simply to calculate the fair market value of their losses and pay them, but intended instead to argue the degree of public liability involved in each separate claim, the English-speaking Honolulu Chamber of Commerce formally protested this action of the administration they had done so much to install and otherwise strongly supported.[30]

Asian claimants opposed the special court even more forcefully. They considered Dole's appointees, in the words of Japanese editor Soga Yasutaro, to be "nothing but second-rate lawyers," in whom Asian leaders had no confidence. Under the special court's guidelines, Japanese and Chinese victims would have to prove the government's liability for the losses they had suffered, as if the issue were being contested between parties in a civil suit, and government lawyers could invoke such factors as zoning violations to reduce the government's liability, thereby punishing Asian residents for negligence on the parts of absentee owners. Asians believed that they had weathered a disproportionately heavy blow in order to save the larger community, and that the larger community should now compensate them for the sacrifice they made, not challenge their right to recompense in an ad hoc courtroom operating under rigged rules.[31]

To help the Dole administration "reflect on the fact that the organization of the claims court lacked justice and fairness," the Provisional Japanese Council, which spoke for Japanese economic interests much as the Chamber of Commerce spoke for white economic interests, decided to approach their counterparts in the Chinese business community. In the words of a participant in this movement, "those of us among the victims were determined by all means to bring about fundamental changes" in the proposed reparations process. Together the community leaders formed the Japanese-Chinese Bi-National United Association, agreed upon a set of resolutions, and then planned a mass meeting to announce them. Newspaper editorials and handbills in three languages publicized that meeting so successfully that it became the largest Asian rally ever held in Honolulu.[32]

Roughly five thousand people, about two-thirds of whom were Chinese, gathered on the grounds of a Japanese school to protest the special court of claims. The flags of China and Japan "were peacefully intertwined" on a temporary stage, and the operative word was "peacefully." Japanese and Chinese businessmen had rarely interacted with one another on terms other than competitive, and ordinary Chinese and Japanese residents had refused only weeks earlier to be intermingled in the quarantine camps. Now the two communities stood together, and their leaders all agreed that it was "a splendid thing to behold." After three hours of oratory in Chinese, Japanese, and English, the completely orderly crowd ratified a resolution denouncing the special court as "unfair and unjust." The resolution passed with a thunderous roar, and not a single dissent was audible. The mass meeting also offered cheers for President McKinley, whose financial backing—if it could be obtained—would offer the merchants their best hope of receiving full compensation, in addition to cheers for China and Japan. A joint committee of seven Chinese leaders and six Japanese leaders agreed to take the protest formally to President Dole.[33]

Faced with a steady litany of editorials denouncing inflated claims, with opposition from his own supporters in the Chamber of Commerce, and now with an unprecedented united front presented by the city's most influential Chinese and Japanese leaders, Dole permanently adjourned his special court of claims the following day, April 9. Like everyone else, he decided to wait for McKinley. In a personal interview with the delegates from the rally, the president vowed "that he would do everything in his power to see to it that the victims would not be subject to any further inconvenience." Dole realized he had made a clumsy mistake, which strengthened the resolve of his opponents, weakened his support in the Chamber of Commerce, inadvertently united the Chinese and Japanese, and turned the reparations issue into a political nightmare.[34]

Even ardent pro-annexationists realized that Dole's mishandling of reparation issues in the short run would make them harder than ever to resolve in the long run. The *Evening Bulletin*, for example, characterized Dole's actions as "a combination expressive of incompetence, ignorance, and poor politics." In the end, the United States government would indeed assume most of the financial burdens of the plague and fire reparations of 1900. But the prolonged and tangled proceedings of the subsequent United States Claims Commission would limp along for years, and despite apparently good intentions, those proceedings would leave a bad taste in the mouths of Hawaiian residents of all races for decades thereafter.[35]

With the prospect of reparations stalled indefinitely, Emerson, Day, and Wood faced rapidly escalating pressures to at least permit the resumption of normal economic activities. They had earlier vowed to keep their policies in effect until thirty days passed without a new case of plague, and because one had occurred on the final day of March, they intended to sustain their emergency measures through April. But restless planters on the outlying islands launched a campaign to end shipping restrictions short of thirty days. Sugar production was a year-round activity in Hawaii, with planting, harvesting, and refining schedules carefully staggered to maximize the productivity of available labor. Since December, those carefully calibrated operations had been on hold, and the planters feared a serious breakdown if they were not soon released from the triumvirate's bans on new labor coming in and refined sugar going out.

The planters were quickly joined by almost all of Honolulu's businessmen, both Asian and English-speaking, whose livelihoods depended directly or indirectly on international commerce. Increasingly vocal merchants pressed the physicians to relinquish their "great executive powers" and to cease their role as "a government within a government—with authority almost exceeding that of a legislature." In the merchants' view, the time had come for the Board of Health to revert to its pre-plague status as a minor agency reporting to the attorney general. The physicians' sharpest critics accused them of prolonging the state of emergency for the sole purpose of continuing to raid the treasury "by use of the plague bugaboo." But Emerson, Day, and Wood refused to bend.[36]

For the Board's physicians, the price of maintaining their policies through April was a constant pummeling from the press. The *Evening Bulletin*, the *Star*, and the *Commercial Advertiser* took turns jabbing the doctors over their ongoing spending, even though plague had disappeared. One of the lowest blows was delivered on April 19, when the *Advertiser* ran a feature story about the way Alexandria, Egypt, had dealt with the plague epidemic. According to the article, the total deaths in Alexandria barely exceeded the total deaths in Honolulu, even though the population of the Egyptian city was estimated to be ten times that of the Hawaiian city. The paper, which had led the cry to burn Chinatown after the death of Sarah Boardman and had floated the possibility of mandatory inoculations, then pointedly observed that Alexandria's sanitary department—in contrast to Honolulu's Board of Health—had achieved its low death rate without recourse to either burning or inoculations. The following day, the *Advertiser* noted smugly that the Alexandria story had been "the subject of much comment on the streets" and had given "impetus to the general feeling among business men" that Emerson, Day, and Wood had pushed their policies far enough.[37]

Tensions came to a head over when and how to begin redevelopment in Chinatown, which had been completely sealed off since late January by a Board-ordered barrier fence. Asian and white businessmen all favored prompt redevelopment. They wanted to believe that *pestis* could not survive very long on its own, and their hopes were buoyed by a report that U.S. surgeon general Wyman submitted to the U.S. Treasury Department. He claimed plague bacilli could not survive more than four hours when exposed to sunlight, more than four days when sitting at room temperature, or more than eight days in sterilized water. If the surgeon general was correct, the businessmen contended, then Chinatown should be clear of contamination by now and rebuilding could safely begin.[38]

But Board physicians still feared the bacilli might be alive in Chinatown's abandoned cesspools or in organic materials below ground. They were also aware that the British in Bombay had not only plowed the ground at plague sites but soaked the soils with petroleum, burned them, and kept the sites isolated for a year. Kitasato was similarly demanding that plague districts in Japan remain vacant for at least a year. Consistent with their approach through the entire crisis, Emerson, Day, and Wood agreed to resolve the impasse by having Hoffman conduct bacteriological surveys of Chinatown's soils. If he did not find plague, the district would be reopened when the plague emergency ended. Hoffman dutifully dug and tested soil samples for the next two weeks, and to the relief of everyone concerned, the samples all came up free of *pestis*.[39]

The triumvirate weathered more criticism when Carmichael lifted all medical restrictions on American military ships bound for the mainland after April 20. Though he had supported his close friends on the Board of Health through the entire crisis, and no doubt would have preferred to support their thirty-day decision, Carmichael was under strong pressure himself. Marine Hospital Service officers exercised a good deal of discretion when it came to assessing local health conditions, and Carmichael knew that it would help him stay on the professional fast track if he expedited the flow of American troops to and from the Philippine Islands, where the United States was fighting Filipino forces in another recently acquired Pacific archipelago. But his action fueled resentment among Honolulu merchants who still had to put up with the expensive and time-consuming inspections, fumigations, and outright bans demanded by their own local physicians, while their new parent government allowed its soldiers to pass through the islands as if plague was no longer a threat. The press, in turn, suggested a public debate over the need to continue the "thirty-day safeguard," and noted the "natural impatience" welling up in the city.[40]

As more days passed without new cases, all parties seemed to soften their positions and prepare for a graceful end to the plague crisis. Though the three physicians maintained strict control over the few people remaining in detention camps, they overlooked technical violations of other quarantine restrictions all around the city. Stores quietly reopened; public amusements resumed; health inspections essentially ceased altogether. In private discussions, the Council of State began to realize how extraordinary the previous five months really had been. Large portions of Honolulu had been burned, the Hawaiian treasury had been drawn down without much accounting or oversight, and the business affairs of the republic were in the hands of three medical professionals who knew nothing about business. Perhaps it was time to reassert their own authority "and try to get back to legal methods."[41]

The *Advertiser*, for its part, stopped hammering the Board of Health and printed a formal tribute to its president, hailing Wood as the man who led the city to victory in "the war waged against plague." No one had ever had so much "power reposed in him," according to the paper, and fortunately for Hawaii, Wood proved himself up to the job. "Though Dr. Wood has a stiff temper and an obstinate will, he possesses also a power of sympathy most invaluable to him as a physician and a man; and though many of his actions during the hight [*sic*] of the plague may have seemed arbitrary and severe to some, yet will the majority acknowledge his sense of justice and sincerity of motive."[42]

The *Advertiser* even ran a follow-up story about Alexandria, Egypt, this time admitting that the death counts officially reported there were meaninglessly low, since most deaths were not officially recorded. The editor also acknowledged that the Egyptian sanitary department had manufactured large supplies of Haffkine's serum and imposed a widespread program of inoculation. Moreover, Alexandria had been forced to maintain its restrictions for an extra six months, not thirty days, as lingering cases

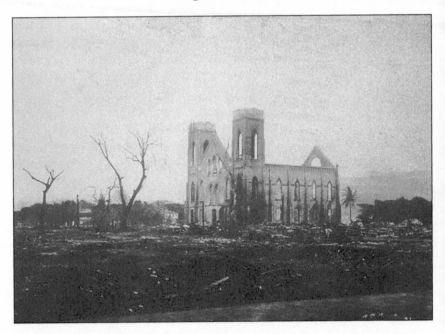

The shell of Kaumakapili Church as it appeared during the cleanup period after the fire. Soon after this picture was taken, the shell was pulled down as a safety precaution. Hawaii State Archives

continued to break out. By those standards, the triumvirate's management of the epidemic in Honolulu was looking magnificent.[43]

On April 27, just three days before all restrictions were due to be lifted, the false rumor of a fresh case of plague spread distress throughout the city. But Board physicians investigated the report and quickly rebutted the story. Three days later the entire Board issued a brief public statement ceremoniously signed by Wood: "I hereby declare the port of Honolulu and all other places in the Hawaiian Islands to be free from infection by bubonic plague. All quarantine regulations adopted by the Board of Health on account of bubonic plague in the Hawaiian Islands are hereby rescinded." The announcement triggered relief and celebration.[44]

14

Aftermath

O n the same day Honolulu Board of Health president Clifford Wood
formally decreed Hawaii free from plague, U.S. president William
McKinley—sitting six thousand miles away in Washington, D.C.—concluded
his morning's work by signing "An Act to Provide a Government for the
Territory of Hawaii," then arose and headed off for lunch. Though weeks
would pass before either man learned of the other's legal action, the day
had produced a remarkable coincidence in Hawaiian history by officially
concluding two interconnected campaigns, one medical and the other
political.[1]

The law McKinley signed granted Hawaii full territorial status under
the Constitution of the United States, thus putting the archipelago on an
equal footing with Arizona, New Mexico, and Oklahoma, which were also
territories at that time. By placing Hawaii on the ultimate path to statehood—
the Senate had rejected a proposal precluding that possibility—the act
culminated the crusade begun eight years before by the annexationists.
Though no one knew it at the time, Hawaii would be the last United
States acquisition to be dealt with in this manner; the other so-called insular possessions gained by the United States at the turn of the twentieth
century, including Puerto Rico, the Philippines, and Guam, never received
the full territorial status afforded to Hawaii. To no one's surprise, McKinley

named Dole as the first territorial governor. For six weeks following the end of the plague emergency, Hawaii returned to civilian rule under the "existing government" and prepared for the transition ahead. On June 14, 1900, amid fireworks and parades, the new territorial government officially came into being.[2]

The federal government also agreed to assume the knotty problem of adjudicating fire claims and paying reparations to people who lost property in the battle to rid the newest American territory of bubonic plague. Since the crisis had occurred during a period of ad hoc government, and since the revenues of the defunct Republic of Hawaii would revert to the new territory anyway, the federal government saw no alternative to providing the money from Washington. The McKinley administration justified the funds on the grounds that the need for "thorough and immediate measures" had been imperative, and the Honolulu Board of Health had properly employed "the usual and approved methods, by fire and otherwise, to stamp out the plague." Although the national government would ordinarily consider any reparations to be the responsibility of the jurisdiction that undertook the destructive actions, Congress decided that the "special and exceptional facts" associated with the transitional government in Hawaii were not likely to recur, and hence that the national government was not setting a precedent for future bailouts, foreign or domestic.[3]

In conjunction with the claims, Congress held hearings about the plague crisis and eventually created a special claims commission. The work of that claims commission was uneven, to say the least. Pending before the commissioners were approximately 6,750 claims totaling almost $3.2 million in requested reparations. At first, the commission began paying the claims approximately at face value. But the commissioners soon began to realize that many of the requests before them were either inflated in various ways or outright frauds, and—at the rate they were initially paying—the money allotted by Congress for this purpose would be gone before all the claims could be considered. Consequently, the commission put the process on hold, then eventually decided to apply what amounted to across-the-board reductions to the vast majority of the remaining claims. In the end, the commissioners awarded slightly under $1.5 million, or somewhat less than half of what people said they actually lost.[4]

Those involved in the claims process found it tremendously frustrating. The paperwork was difficult and all forms had to be filed in English or Hawaiian, so most claimants were forced to hire lawyers. The proceedings themselves were tedious and time-consuming. The commissioners challenged people to remember specific details—exact prices to the penny, for example—that they could not always recall with crystal accuracy, yet the same commissioners refused to admit into evidence such tangible items as charred bundles of paper money with their denominations still barely legible. Even when their claims were partly successful, most claimants did not receive a cent from the U.S. government until 1903, long after they had been forced to start over on their own.[5]

Under Consul Saito, Japanese residents who lost property to the plague fires organized the Japanese Victims Representation Committee to act as a central clearinghouse and advocacy group. The Victims Committee worked to minimize the degree of inflation in Japanese claims, an effort that produced hard feelings within the community. At the local level, Saito toiled tirelessly for his constituents and eventually convinced the Japanese government in Tokyo to press the United States government in Washington on behalf of their countrymen in Hawaii. Even the Chinese admired Saito's energy, and—probably as a veiled criticism of their own consul—they praised Saito's wholehearted commitment to all of the Japanese in Honolulu. Moreover, the Japanese had largely supported the triumvirate's approach to fighting the plague and had accepted life in the quarantine camps with remarkable grace.[6]

In the final reckoning, however, the Japanese as a group received just slightly more than half the total face value of the claims they submitted. Though this turned out to be a higher percentage than any other group of claimants received, thousands of Japanese people who had been forced to sacrifice for the common good of the entire city found themselves having to start over with little or nothing in the wake of the plague crisis.

Among Chinese, the claims process left bitter and long-lasting animosities. Many of the claims paid at face value early in the process had been from Chinese businessmen allied with Consul Yang, and even Chinese sources conceded that the commissioners were right to suspect that some of those claims had been fraudulently inflated. The United Chinese Society tried to improve the situation by establishing their own claims-clearing office, and by urging people to base their requests strictly "on the truth" because falsehoods and errors would delay the process for everyone. "Every society member," they admonished, "has the duty to evaluate [claims] based on justice and reality." When the society's officers felt a claim was fraudulent, they returned it and told the victim to pursue reparations on his own without the support of the society.[7]

But the federal claims commission could not make legal distinctions between claims reviewed by the United Chinese Society and inflated claims submitted independently. As a practical matter, the commissioners contin-ued to apply their de facto discount to all of them. Consequently, many claimants who tried to cooperate with the United Chinese Society came away feeling cheated not only by the United States government, which ar-bitrarily reduced their losses, but also by duplicitous fellow Chinese who submitted inflated claims and who in many cases were also their political opponents. Kong Tai Heong believed that some of the hatred directed in later years at her and her husband, Li Khai Fai, stemmed not from the plague crisis per se but from efforts by others in the Chinese community to channel resentment away from themselves. Some Chinese, she told her daughter, had actually been "happy that there had been a fire. But they tried to hide their happiness by piling blame on father [for reporting plague cases in the first place], hoping this would help hide the fat gains they had made from the parched bones of those who had lost their goods in the fire."[8]

Most Chinese, like most Japanese, received some recompense, but far less than they deserved. Chung Kun Ai, for example, received enough money for the loss of City Mill to repay his company's debts, but the commissioners awarded him only a small portion of the value of his per-sonal property. He thus found himself back in the position he had been in before launching City Mill, rather than in the position he had achieved as director of a multinational business. Many other Chinese, forced to start over with nothing, fared far worse.[9]

A committee of five Chinese claimants in December 1902 reminded the American government that on the day of the great fire the people of Chinatown had accepted assurances that they would be compensated for their losses. But two years had passed, and many of the former refugees were still "forced to live upon public and private charity." According to the committee, "many of the sufferers became despondent and were led to take their own lives; others worried over their losses so much, wonder-ing whether they would ever regain their former standing in the commu-nity which years of unremitting toil had established, that it brought on sickness and death, leaving their wives and children in helpless circum-stances; and still others were driven to insanity."[10]

Looking back from the 1920s, an anonymous Chinese writer who was otherwise pro-American nonetheless reminded his readers—in a compre-hensive survey of the Chinese in Hawaii—that rebuilding a business "was not an easy task, and Chinese businesses suffered irreparable losses [dur-ing the plague crisis]. . . . It was not easy to rally one's forces after a de-feat." A full seventy years after the great fire, the historian Tin-Yuke Char observed, "Even today, when one talks with members of the older generation whose families lost their belongings and went through quarantine and fumigation, one learns that it was an emotionally scarring experience for people who found it difficult to hold the authorities blameless." In the early years of the twenty-first century, Honolulu's most prominent local historian still characterized the fire of 1900 as "the holocaust of Honolulu Chinatown" and alleged the secret murder of Chinese residents in the guise of fighting plague. In that view, the entire process looked like a deliberate act of racist revenge, planned far in advance by Lorrin Thurston in retaliation against the Chinese merchants who helped Robert Wilcox try to unseat the annexationists in 1895.[11]

It would be wrong, however, to see relations between the races in Honolulu as completely adversarial after the plague crisis. Even though the burned-out blocks of Chinatown represented prime real estate in a superb commercial location—potentially more valuable than ever with its shabby structures completely removed—the territorial government resisted intense pressures from white developers to resettle Chinatown residents elsewhere in the city and turn the burned-out blocks over to white businesses. Instead, the city installed modern water systems and sanitary sewers at public expense, while prior owners and residents rebuilt—usually with brick and stone this time—and returned. Unfortunately, that process also bred confusion, litigation, and hard bargains, because the city had to realign some of Chinatown's preexisting streets to accommodate the sanitary improvements. For every shift, even if only a few feet, lot lines had to be redrawn to preserve street-front access—a complicated process that led to extended haggling.

Partly as a result of the remapping, partly because new sanitary laws and tenement regulations forced the district to be rebuilt less densely than it had formerly been, and partly to escape a place that had brought them so much misery, many Asians moved away from the Chinatown district to other areas of Honolulu during the first decade of the twentieth century. Nonetheless, many Asian businesses were able to relocate essentially where they had been before the plague fires, including perhaps most symbolically the Wing Wo Tai company, where the death of bookkeeper You Chong had signaled arrival of the world epidemic. Renovated again in 1979, the Wing Wo Tai building still stands on Nuuanu Street today. Kaumakapili's twin spires have been replaced by a soaring pair of luxury high-rise apartments—secular twin spires in their own right—and the Nimitz Highway cuts through an area where Chinese produce markets did business in 1899. But the core of the area destroyed in the great fire of 1900 remains "Chinatown" to the present time—and continues to house a variety of ethnic, racial, and linguistic groups, including a growing number of Vietnamese businesses.[12]

Soga Yasutaro, the junior editor who saved *Hawaii Shimpo*'s printing press and escaped from the Kalihi detention camp, noted two other positive legacies of the plague and fire crisis. One was the willingness of Honolulu's Chinese and Japanese leaders to cooperate for mutually desirable goals. From their joint reparations protest and the Asian mass meeting emerged the Japanese-Chinese Federation. Soga acknowledged that relations between the two groups did not change overnight—he lightheartedly joked that the grandly named federation sometimes consisted of him and a Chinese friend out drinking, and he noted that the federation had trouble getting its members to pay dues. But he also rightly recognized that the organization provided a forum during the first decades of the twentieth century that led to higher levels of Asian cooperation under the new territorial government than had existed under the republic.

The other positive result that Soga recalled was the inadvertent "cleaning up of Honolulu's downtown Japanese underworld." "Prostitutes and gangsters," he believed, "feared that the authorities would extend their post-fire consolidation and disposal to them as well, and they decided to scatter to the four winds." Whether that was altogether the case is hard to judge, but the transitional government did make a concerted effort in May to prevent the reestablishment of Japanese brothels. Later police figures also suggested that Japanese criminal activity declined in Honolulu and rose on Maui, which was where Soga thought many of the city's least savory Japanese residents had fled.[13]

Soga himself remained in the newspaper business in Honolulu, where he took over the *Yamato Shimbun* in 1905, renamed it the *Nippu Jiji*, and turned it into the most widely read Japanese paper in the islands. After backing the strikers in a famous plantation labor dispute in 1909, Soga served four months in jail for conspiracy before returning home to a hero's welcome. He lived long enough to be summarily arrested the night Japan attacked Pearl Harbor and be interned for a third time by Americans at various World War II relocation camps in Hawaii and on the mainland. Again welcomed back to Honolulu when the war was over, he continued on as one of the revered fathers of Japanese-American journalism until his death in 1957.[14]

At least some degree of business cooperation between whites and Asians survived the economic devastation of the fires. Chung Kun Ai, who initially assumed that the fire had finished him as an entrepreneur, was able to reestablish City Mill because white companies agreed to advance him materials at cost and consciously decided not to press him for regular payments, even though they could have foreclosed on his assets. The white law firm that renegotiated City Mill's contracts and handled Chung's claims before the commission charged less than a quarter of what its fees had been prior to the fire. As Chung put it plainly, "They [the white businesses and law firms] chose not to profit from City Mill's disaster."

Such relations may not have been the norm. Most of the prestigious white law firms representing Asian claimants before the claims commission charged 6.5 percent of whatever they recovered. Though treated well himself, Chung heard about a lawyer "who swallowed up every cent he could from [other] poor fire-sufferers." Chung's earlier conversion to Christianity almost certainly helped him establish trust with white businessmen, as Christianity had done for Vice-Consul Gu as well. Nonetheless, such acts of good will did take place, and Chung Kun Ai went on to become a leading business figure in Honolulu. He eventually established a charitable foundation of his own to help others as he had been helped, and he continued to expand City Mill, which today is run by his grandson and employs some 450 people.[15]

Many of the relief societies established during the plague crisis remained intact and continued to contribute to the welfare of Honolulu. The Japanese Aid Society built a Japanese hospital in the wake of the plague crisis, as the Chinese had done in the wake of the cholera crisis. Within six months of the great fire, enough money had been raised to build a thirty-eight-bed facility in the Kapalama district. Mori Iga, one of the physicians who had worked closely and cooperatively with Emerson, Day, and Wood through the plague period, served as the hospital's first director. Following several stages of expansion, a number of relocations, and a new name, that small Japanese Charity Hospital eventually emerged as Honolulu's modern Kuakini Hospital and Health System, now open to all Honolulu residents.[16]

Emerson, Day, and Wood, the three physicians whose five months of absolute rule had been among the most eventful in Hawaii's history, returned to their private lives and all but disappeared from public view. As soon as the plague crisis was over, Day took his wife on a trip around the world that lasted more than two years. For Day, the trip was partly a journey of relief and reward after five months of battling *pestis* night and day, and partly a great adventure while he could still enjoy traveling. When the couple returned to Honolulu, Day rejoined the medical partnership he had formed in 1899 with his boyhood pal Wood and resumed his practice from their mutual offices on Beretania Street. But Day—the doctor who had left Chicago for his health in 1886—was never again robust after the plague crisis. He died in 1906 at the age of 46.[17]

Emerson, the aging "mission boy" and veteran public health officer, resumed his medical practice in Honolulu, but spent increasing amounts of his time on literary, historical, and linguistic pursuits. Ever purposeful and fit, he also swam every morning in the ocean. Though he declined any additional government appointments, he served as president of several civic, social, and professional organizations, including the Hawaiian Historical Society. Emerson's translation of David Malo's master work on Hawaiian mythology and folklore was published by the U.S. Bureau of Ethnology in 1909, and Emerson's own magnum opus on Hawaiian culture—the product of seven years of research—appeared in 1915, the same year he died in Honolulu at the age of 76.[18]

Wood remained the most prominent of the three in the medical profession. When the Dole administration's Board of Health was replaced by the new United States Territorial Board of Health, Wood was appointed to serve on it. In 1904, he and his wife toured the major hospitals of Europe. Shortly after his return to Honolulu, he helped open Kauikeolani Children's Hospital. Following the death of his friend and partner Day, Wood remained in active practice by himself and served at various times as an officer and principal promoter for Queen's Hospital, as a champion of the Red Cross, as a member and president of the revamped Hawaiian Territorial Medical Association, and as chairman of the Territorial Board of Medical Examiners. He died in Honolulu in 1939 at the age of 79.[19]

Hoffman, the city bacteriologist who bravely performed more than two hundred autopsies during the plague crisis and tried unsuccessfully to develop an antidote to the disease, took the bride he had married in the midst of the emergency on a trip back to Berlin in 1901 to see his homeland and meet his family. The couple returned to Honolulu and lived there until 1910, when they left to resettle permanently in Chicago, where his wife had been raised. To secure an American practice, Hoffman decided to pursue another medical degree. He chose Rush Medical College, where his Honolulu friends Day and Wood had both studied. Hoffman then practiced pediatrics in Chicago, where for many years he was on the staff of Children's Memorial and Presbyterian Hospital. He died in 1945 at the age of 72.[20]

Carmichael, the U.S. Marine Hospital Service physician who had worked so closely with Emerson, Day, and Wood, remained in that federal agency, which would soon enlarge its purview and change its name to the U.S. Public Health Service. In April 1901 he was transferred to San

Francisco to help that city cope with the same pandemic of bubonic plague he had just been battling in Honolulu. But the San Francisco assignment went badly from the outset. Carmichael's marriage, which had come unglued in Honolulu, ended completely when his wife—claiming physical abuse—sued him for divorce only months after arriving on the mainland. As a federal medical officer, he found himself involved in nasty political confrontations with state and local officials. Carmichael had been on the fast track when he arrived in Honolulu a year ahead of the plague, but the ugly infighting in San Francisco derailed his career. The Public Health Service all but exiled him in 1902 to a permanent station on the island of Martha's Vineyard, where he lived the rest of his life. A rather lonely and tragic figure thereafter, Carmichael remained single until the age of 72, when he married for the third time. He died in 1929 at the age of 77.[21]

While the principal policy makers faded from public view as individuals, their collective actions during the plague crisis have been the subject of assessment and disagreement for more than a hundred years. The most damning charge against them, that the Chinatown fire of January 20, 1900, was an intentional act, can be laid to rest. Though some people alleged a conspiracy at the time, and variations of their accusations have continued to serve social, economic, and political purposes ever since, eyewitnesses at the time testified from many different positions and in many different languages that the great fire itself was unintentional. Vice-Consul Gu, the United Chinese Society, the *Tanshan Longji Xi Bao* [Hawaiian Chinese News], and others writing in Chinese; editor Soga and others writing in Japanese; the *Ke Aloha Aina* and others writing in Hawaiian; and literally hundreds of English-language accounts, including accounts from inveterate critics of the Dole administration, all agreed. The surprise wind shifts on January 20 were unusual and could not have been predicted; the fire department tried heroically to contain the fire; and the authorities on all sides were stunned by what happened. When pressed for evidence to the contrary by two U.S. senators in 1903, even Robert Wilcox, the man who had led an armed insurrection against Dole's republic in 1895 and had gone to Washington in 1901 as spokesman for the Home Rule Party, admitted that charges of conscious intent were no more than hearsay and rumor.[22]

More difficult to assess was the decision to use fire in the first place. Even if they did not intend to destroy Chinatown in one great conflagration, Emerson, Day, and Wood were clearly prepared to burn the entire district piecemeal if plague kept occurring there. The three physicians believed from the outset, to repeat the words of their president, that "plague [was] preeminently a disease of locality and place." In the long run, they thought, "The place is much more dangerous than the person," so the place would have to be purged of *pestis*. Moreover, they were vehemently determined from the outset to make sure plague was not merely checked, but "entirely stamped out" in Honolulu, so the disease could not "recur again next year or any time." In that, they shared Lorrin Thurston's long-standing and often-repeated nightmare that went back at least as far as the leprosy controversies: the future prospects of everyone in the archipelago were "doomed" if Hawaii became "known as a plague spot." Consequently, according to their own explanation, "after careful consideration" and "free discussion in open meetings," the physicians "chose fire as the surest and most thorough and most expeditious" method of assuring their goal. Fire and only fire, they assured a subcommittee of U.S. senators in 1902, "would destroy the plague germs."[23]

For that decision the physicians on the Honolulu Board of Health were much admired by their contemporaries elsewhere around the world. Less than two weeks after the great fire, the San Francisco Board of Health, facing its own threat of plague, sent "a special representative" to Hawaii to assess firsthand the actions being taken by their Honolulu counterparts. That representative, Ichitaro Katsuki, was a Japanese-born physician who had graduated from the University of California Medical School and had practiced in San Francisco since 1896. Katsuki applauded the campaign being waged by the Board doctors in Honolulu, joined them in their bacteriological investigations, and worked actively with them in their laboratory searches for a plague serum. He especially admired "the coolness and intelligence which the [Honolulu Board of Health] has manifested." "Honolulu," he continued, "deserves the warm commendation and thanks of every community for its magnificent efforts in coping with the disease."[24]

Unlike the emissary from their city's Board of Health, Chinese residents back in San Francisco itself drew entirely different conclusions. They were well informed about the events in Honolulu, and for them the Hawaiian Board's actions demonstrated the ways in which policies promulgated in the name of public health, especially when implemented without regard to larger contexts, could produce disastrous consequences. As a result, San Francisco's Chinese were on guard against the possibility of something like the Chinatown fire occurring in their city, with its long and violent history of anti-Asian activity. Just as the Chinese expected, an outbreak of plague in San Francisco's Chinatown in March 1900 prompted members of both the San Francisco Board of Health and the California State Board of Health to cite what they regarded as the remarkable success of their counterparts in Honolulu and to begin calling for the burning of San Francisco's Chinatown. Led by the so-called Six Companies, the Chinese immediately countered by hiring top American law firms to defend their rights successfully in court under the Fourteenth Amendment. They also negotiated with the San Francisco Board of Health to implement alternative measures short of burning.[25]

While the Chinese of San Francisco saw the plague crisis in Honolulu as reinforcing the need for caution and restraint, international public health officers almost universally shared Katsuki's point of view. All around the world during the first decade of the twentieth century, public health officers repeatedly hailed the impressive victory of the Honolulu Board of Health under tough and dangerous circumstances. The triumvirate's strong policy of removing survivors to safe ground and then burning the sites of infection left behind had worked: a major infestation of *pestis* was defeated, and no one was killed in the bacteria-destroying conflagrations, even the one that got out of hand. In particular, the fact that no one died of plague in any of the detention camps seemed powerful proof to international public health officers that the fundamental assumptions of the Honolulu physicians had been right all along.[26]

The sentiments of William J. Galbraith, chief surgeon to the Union Pacific Railroad, were typical of many others. "I consider the manner in which the plague trouble has been met in Honolulu," he stated, "as unique in the history of the world," and the "heroic measures" taken by the three "conscientious, up-to-date, and skillful physicians" will produce "immense benefits to future generations." Joseph J. Kinyoun, a pioneer public health officer who had headed the first bacteriological laboratory established by the Marine Hospital Service in 1887 (a laboratory that evolved into the National Institutes of Health) and who had fought the plague pandemic of the 1890s from Hong Kong to San Francisco, strongly agreed with that opinion. Kinyoun believed that the Honolulu triumvirate had at last provided "civilized communities" everywhere with a successful formula for beating *pestis*, provided they had the wherewithal to apply it. He envied the "fortunate circumstances" that had allowed the three Honolulu doctors to act so boldly. Given the resistance he faced at his post in San Francisco to policies like those implemented in Honolulu, he feared that plague might never be eradicated from San Francisco.[27]

Consequently, far from seeing the great Chinatown fire in Honolulu as a sobering reason to avoid site burning, plague fighters around the world often added fire to the weapons they used after 1900. In Kobe, Japan, in 1901, Kitasato, who had been elevated to the post of director of the Imperial Japanese Institute for the Study of Infectious Diseases, implemented essentially the same fire policy that the Honolulu Board had used the previous year, though he was less generous about letting people return to former plague neighborhoods. International public health protocols adopted in Berlin in 1902 all but codified the Honolulu model for dealing with plague. Mexican public health physicians employed site burning when the pandemic reached Mazatlán in 1903. Both Russian and Chinese public health officers burned plague sites in Manchuria in 1910. At least through 1907, official guidelines of the U.S. Public Health Service still insisted that "buildings in which plague continues to manifest itself after [attempted disinfection] should be vacated and destroyed to prevent the spread of the disease."[28]

Looking back in 1904, Kinyoun also believed that the Honolulu Board of Health had done better than any other health board in the world at overcoming the commercial greed of their local businessmen and the selfish defenses of local property holders. The Honolulu physicians' extraordinary emergency powers, in Kinyoun's view, had allowed them to act exclusively for the common good and place the long-term health of their city ahead of any short-term economic considerations. Kinyoun knew personally just how hard that could be: in 1901 he had been removed from his duties as commander of the federal government's San Francisco Quarantine Station following open confrontations with San Francisco businessmen, both white and Chinese, over how to deal with the threat of plague in that city.[29]

The nearly unanimous praise from public health officials around the world helps bring into focus one of the profound ironies of this tale: the policies that produced the great Chinatown fire in Honolulu were not aberrations; they resulted from good-faith efforts on the part of Emerson, Day, and Wood to implement what seemed to them to be the most progressive public health ideas of their time. While they surely acted within—and were influenced by—racist assumptions and territorial ambitions, the three physicians appear from the perspective of the early twenty-first century to have responded to the pandemic of the late nineteenth century first and foremost as medical professionals. On the one hand, that suggests the optimistic possibility that professional commitments, professional training, and professional ethics can—sometimes and to some extent—begin to mitigate the racial and imperial dynamics of their times; on the other hand, it makes clear that even what appear to be the best and most progressive of professional commitments are sometimes capable of producing unforeseen consequences of tragic proportions, especially in situations where the knowledge base upon which they rest is shaky and especially in situations where few checks of any other kind are in place. And that is one of the most sobering aspects of this entire incident.

Consider the role of race in these policies. Certainly the Dole administration for which the Board physicians worked was an overtly racist regime, and certainly the fact that Honolulu's poorest slum was overwhelmingly inhabited by Asians and Hawaiians was related to the racist policies of that and preceding governments. Just as certainly, Emerson, Day, and Wood harbored many of the racist assumptions typical of their class and era. Wood, the Board president, later remarked to a congressional committee that the residents of Chinatown at the time of the plague crisis "wallowed in [filth] as only Asiatics can and live." But the triumvirate's actual policies seem to have been neither motivated primarily by race nor implemented in a consciously racist manner. They did not quarantine Honolulu's Chinese, Japanese, or Hawaiian populations in general; they quarantined that minority of the city's Chinese, Japanese, and Hawaiian residents who lived in the infected area from which they feared plague was most likely to spread. They did not burn only those buildings where nonwhites contracted plague; they burned all buildings associated with plague cases, including white homes and major businesses. As Carmichael reported to the surgeon general in Washington, "The sanitary fires were numerous, and the dwellings of Caucasians and Asiatics were treated alike when condemned as foci of infection."[30]

Even more significantly, the Board consistently blocked the far more overtly racist desires of the Citizens' Sanitary Commission, of many white businessmen, and of the traditional physicians in their own medical community, all of whom were calling for the widespread incineration of any areas around the city that appeared to them to be less orderly and, in their minds, potentially less healthy than prim white neighborhoods. Instead, and against heavy pressure, the Board stuck to its policy that bacteriologically confirmed plague sites would be the only ones destroyed, and it refused to authorize preemptive strikes. Under the chaotic and genuinely frightening circumstances that prevailed in the face of bubonic plague, that commitment to policies they regarded as scientifically defensible took genuine political and personal courage. In this regard, the physicians on the Board were forces of professional logic and restraint in the face of irrational fears and prejudices. The irony, of course, lay in the accident of the great fire, which summarily accomplished in one day exactly the kind of outcome those who were willing to act on overtly racist propensities had been seeking.

Though difficult to judge, imperial pressures on the three physicians may have influenced their actions more strongly than racial pressures. All of the principals involved in determining and executing the Board's policies from the beginning of the antiplague campaign had strongly favored the annexation of Hawaii to the United States, and all fervently hoped for the consummation of full territorial status. Since that status was still in doubt when the world plague epidemic hit Honolulu, the three physicians urgently wanted to avoid the impression that Hawaii was too plague ridden to merit a traditional territorial government. Put differently, they might not have moved so aggressively toward the rapid deployment of their most destructive weapon if Hawaii had not been under intense scrutiny by Congress but had instead already achieved American territorial status.

Adding to the imperial pressures was the fear of looking like a government incapable of maintaining its own public health. Recently installed imperial powers tend to move aggressively against threats to public health, as the United States was doing in the Philippines (against cholera) and in Panama (against yellow fever) at roughly this same time and as China did (against avian flu) as recently as 1997, when that nation had just repossessed Hong Kong. Indeed, China's vigorous and self-consciously visible response to avian flu in Hong Kong stood in sharp contrast to that same government's initially defensive and almost clandestine handling of the SARS epidemic in its own heartland five years later. Consciously or unconsciously, such shows of medical force in recently acquired areas demonstrate the power of the new authorities and stake a claim to the sanction of beneficent rule.[31]

The United States had just annexed Hawaii when the plague struck, and the Dole administration was still a shaky regime in search of legitimacy. As a result, the Board of Health was under heavy psychological pressure to act dramatically. Local critics of the Dole administration intuitively recognized those pressures and sarcastically noted that medical and governmental "coincidences are strange bedfellows: Cholera and revolution in 1895, and plague and territorial government in 1899–1900." Moreover, members of the Honolulu Board of Health were well aware that publications such as the Boston *Herald*, a newspaper opposed to territorial status for Hawaii, were complaining that the United States would be forced to send "a medical despot" out to restore the archipelago's public health, an accusation the Board's physicians wanted—perhaps too fervently—to refute. Still, by themselves, the territorial aspirations and imperial visions of the Dole administration cannot fully account for the triumvirate's behavior.[32]

In the end, the policies implemented by Emerson, Day, and Wood are probably best understood as the logical consequence of their professional commitment to a bacteriological understanding of disease, combined with incomplete bacteriological knowledge and an absence of bacteriological weapons with which to fight that disease. Fortunately, both a better understanding of the disease and alternative weapons for fighting it would develop shortly. As a consequence, site burning died out quite quickly as a major tactic against plague epidemics. Its last systematic use in the United States appears to have taken place in Los Angeles in 1924. When plague broke out in a Mexican section of the city, local health officials employed quarantine and destruction methods similar to those used in Honolulu in 1900. But when the U.S. Public Health Service stepped in and assumed control of the situation in Los Angeles, that federal agency suspended the policy, declaring that the fires per se would have little practical effect.[33]

With a century's hindsight, Honolulu's battle against bubonic plague appears to have been among the most incandescent events in what might be characterized as a brief and rather ironic "heroic age" of bacteriologically based public health. Fire was strong medicine, but it was the only medicine then available that was known with absolute certainty to kill *pestis* and hence purge a given area of what was thought to be entrenched disease. As an endorser of the Board's fire policy acknowledged on the day after the city's first burning, "This is heroic treatment, but it is a policy which gives assurance of victory which no other does." Embedded in and influenced by a context of intense racial and imperial pressures—and completely unrestrained by ordinary civilian procedures—Emerson, Day, and Wood decided to prescribe that medicine.[34]

In the final analysis, such distinctions—though useful in considering the sobering lessons of the Chinatown fire in the history of public health—probably mattered little to the residents of Chinatown at the time. Thousands of people had lived for months in fear of contracting bubonic plague, wondered for weeks whether they would lose all of the material gains they worked so hard under such difficult circumstances to accumulate, staggered through a terrifying day of trauma as their neighborhoods burned around them, put up with incarceration in temporary camps, and then had to start over with long-delayed and unfair compensation for the sacrifices imposed upon them for the common good by a government that excluded their participation. For them, the battle against bubonic plague and the burning of Chinatown were devastating episodes they would never forget.

Notes

ABBREVIATIONS

AHW	*Austin's Hawaiian Weekly* (Honolulu)
BHM	*Bulletin of the History of Medicine*
BMA	Bishop Museum Library and Archives, Honolulu
EBU	*Evening Bulletin* (Honolulu)
FRI	*Friend* (Honolulu)
HGZ	*Hawaiian Gazette* (Honolulu)
HBH	Honolulu Board of Health Files, Hawaii State Archives, Honolulu
HHS	Hawaiian Historical Society, Honolulu
HIN	Subcommittee on Pacific Islands and Porto [*sic*] Rico, *Hawaiian Investigation*, 57th Congress (Washington, D.C., 1903)
HJH	*Hawaiian Journal of History*
HMC	Hawaiian Mission Children's Society Library, Honolulu
HSA	Hawaii State Archives, Honolulu
HUN	Henry E. Huntington Library and Art Gallery, San Marino, California
IND	*Independent* (Honolulu)

JHM   *Journal of the History of Medicine and Allied Sciences*

KAA   *Ke Aloha Aina* (Honolulu)

MAM   Mamiya Medical Heritage Center, Archives and Medical Museum, Hawaii Medical Library, Honolulu

MBH   "Minutes of the Board of Health," 1899–1900 (typescript), Hawaii State Archives, Honolulu

MHS   Marine Hospital Service, Correspondence Files, RG 90, Archives II, Adelphi, Maryland

NLM   History of Medicine Division, National Library of Medicine, Bethesda, Maryland

PCA   *Pacific Commercial Advertiser* (Honolulu)

PHS   Office of the Chief Historian, United States Public Health Service, Rockville, Maryland

YS   *Yamato Shimbun* (Honolulu)

ACKNOWLEDGMENTS

1. I have made many inquiries about that sign over several years. While people sometimes remember seeing it, I have been unable to find anyone who knew exactly why it disappeared. People I talked to at the Hawaiian Chinese History Society, the Chinese Chamber of Commerce, and the United Chinese Society were unable to discover who put the sign up or why it came down. I once discussed the sign with the daughter of the honorable Hiram Fong, who in turn raised the question with her father. But they were likewise unable to find out what happened. James Ho, Chinatown's leading local historian and curator of the district's historical museum, surmised that the sign almost certainly fell victim to one of the major building renewal projects of the 1980s, but even he could not recall who had erected it or why it was never replaced.

PROLOGUE

1. MBH, January 20, 1900, 189.

CHAPTER 1

1. For an excellent overview of this pandemic, see Myron Echenberg, "Pestis Redux: The Initial Years of the Third Bubonic Plague Pandemic, 1894–1901," *Journal of World History*, Vol. 13, No. 2 (2002), 429–49, which also contains

footnotes to the growing literature on this plague; and Carol Benedict, *Bubonic Plague in Nineteenth-Century China* (Stanford, 1996).

2. Li Ling Ai, *Life Is for a Long Time: A Chinese Hawaiian Memoir* (New York, 1972), 19; W. J. Simpson, *Report on the Causes and Continuance of Plague in Hongkong and Suggestions as to Remedial Measures* (London, 1903); M. D. Regan, *The Whitewash Brigade: The Hong Kong Plague of 1894* (London, 1998).

3. On the symptoms of bubonic plague, see Paul D. Hoeprich et al., *Infectious Diseases* (Philadelphia, 1994), 1302–12; Sherwood L. Gorbach et al., *Infectious Diseases* (Philadelphia, 1998), 1568–75; and Gerald L. Mandell et al., *Principles and Practice of Infectious Diseases* (New York, 2000), 2406–14.

4. Roy Porter, *The Greatest Benefit to Mankind: A Medical History of Humanity* (New York, 1997) and Irvine Loudon, ed., *Western Medicine* (New York, 1997) are recent summaries of the long-standard position that the plague of the 1890s was the same bubonic plague that caused the black death and subsequent pandemics. The World Health Organization (WHO) currently recognizes three historic periods of plague: the Justinian (sixth to eighth centuries); the black death (fourteenth to eighteenth centuries); and the contemporary (ca. 1860 to the present). By making no distinctions among the three, WHO implies that the same disease caused them all. Recently, however, Samuel K. Cohn Jr. has amassed impressive evidence that the bubonic plague of the Middle Ages and the bubonic plague of modern times may have produced similar symptoms but could not reasonably have been the same disease. See Samuel K. Cohn Jr., "The Black Death: End of a Paradigm," *American Historical Review*, Vol. 107, No. 3 (June 2002), 703–38, and Cohn, *The Black Death Transformed: Disease and Culture in Early Renaissance Europe* (London and New York, 2002). Medical literature suggests that bubonic plague is capable of mutating quite rapidly into variant strains. See, for example, Guiyoule et al., "Recent Emergence of New Variants of *Yersinia Pestis* in Madagascar," *Journal of Clinical Microbiology*, Vol. 35 (November 1997), 2826–33, and Perry and Fetherston, "*Yersinia Pestis*—Etiological Agent of Plague," *Clinical Microbiology Review*, Vol. 10 (January 1997), 35–66.

5. David J. Bibel and T. H. Chen, "Diagnosis of Plague: an Analysis of the Yersin-Kitasato Controversy," *Bacteriological Reviews*, Vol. 40, No. 3 (September 1976), 633–51; Norman Howard-Jones, "Kitasato, Yersin, and the Plague Bacillus," *Clio Medica*, Vol. 10, No 1 (1975), 23–27; Paul Hauduroy, "Comment Alexandre Yersin decouvrit le microbe de la peste," *Yersin et la peste* (Lausanne, 1944); James R. Bartholomew, "The Acculturation of Science in Japan: Kitasato Shibasaburo and the Japanese Bacteriological Community, 1885–1920" (Ph.D. diss., Stanford, 1971); Edward Marriott, *The Plague Race: A Tale of Fear, Science, and Heroism* (London, 2002). Yersin's strain was subsequently determined to be the actual cause of the disease.

6. "Microbe of the Plague, magnified 20,000 diameters," and the story about Yersin in *PCA*, December 16, 1899; see also *EBU*, December 12, 1899.

7. For an excellent discussion of this process and the epidemiological impact of different flea species in spreading plague, see Marilyn Chase, *The Barbary Plague: The Black Death in Victorian San Francisco* (New York, 2003),188–91. The flea vector was strongly suspected from 1904 onward, and finally proven by the British Commission for the Investigation of Plague in India. See also Robert Barde, "Prelude to the Plague: Public Health and Politics at America's Pacific Gateway, 1899," *JHM*, Vol. 58, No. 2 (April 2003), 153–86; Mary P. Sutphen, "Not What, but Where: Bubonic Plague and the Reception of Germ Theories in Hong Kong and Calcutta, 1894–1897," *JHM*, Vol. 52, No. 1 (January 1997), 81–113.

8. Simpson, *Report on the Causes,* especially p. 8; Walter Wyman, *The Bubonic Plague* (Washington, D.C., 1900). Wyman had been publishing versions of these arguments elsewhere since at least 1896. A. Shadwell, "The Plague in Oporto," *Nineteenth Century,* Vol. XLVI (July–December 1899), 846. For evidence of persistent confusion on the subject of rats and plague, even among well-informed physicians, see an undated letter from James J. Molony to Clifford B. Wood about the death of a Chinese passenger aboard a ship. Molony served as the ship's doctor during this period. Molony File, MAM; C. Marsh-Beadnell, "The Prevention of Bubonic Plague," *British Medical Journal* (1904), 1133. For public confusion in Honolulu, see "Some Notes on Plague," *AHW* (December 16, 1899), 3.

9. Ann Marcovich, "French Colonial Medicine and Colonial Rule: Algeria and Indochina," in Roy Macleod and Milton Lewis, eds., *Disease, Medicine, and Empire: Perspectives on Western Medicine and the Experience of European Expansion* (London and New York, 1988), 103–17; Radhika Ramasubban, "Imperial Health in British India, 1857–1900," in Macleod and Lewis, pp. 38–60. See among many examples: A. K. Chalmers, "Actions Taken at Glasgow to Stamp Out Plague," *Public Health* [New York], (December 1900), 183–87, and "Directions for Combating Plague," forwarded to Washington, D.C., by the U.S. consul-general in Berlin and later reprinted in *United States Public Health Reports,* Vol. 17, part 2 (1902), 2371–73. "Report on the International Sanitary Conference Held at Venice (February 16 to March 19, 1897)," *United States Public Health Reports,* Vol. 12 (1897), 452–59. On the international politics of quarantine during the nineteenth century, see Peter Baldwin, *Contagion and the State in Europe, 1830–1930* (Cambridge, 1999).

10. Guenter Risse, "No Burning: Race, Public Health and Civil Rights in San Francisco's Chinatown, 1900," paper presented at the Policy History Conference, St. Louis, Mo., May 31, 2002.

11. "Stop the Asiatics," *AHW* (January 20, 1900), 1; "The Grim Visitor," *AHW* (December 16, 1899), 2; *IND,* December 13, 1899, p. 3; Anna Leadingham to unknown, n.d. [ca. December 30, 1899, on the basis of internal evidence], Manuscript Collections, HHS.

12. Clarence E. Glick, *Sojourners and Settlers: Chinese Migrants in Hawaii* (Honolulu, 1980), table 10, p. 128.
13. U.S. Bureau of the Census, *Twelfth Census of the United States*, Vol. 1 (Washington, D.C., 1901), 613; Andrew W. Lind, *Hawaii's People* (Honolulu, 1967), 50. Honolulu was in the process of taking a city census of its own when the plague struck. For preliminary reports of that tally, see *FRI*, Vol. 58, No. 2 (February 1900). An excellent indication of urban sprawl can be gained from "Map of Honolulu Showing Progress of Sewer Construction, 1899–1900," opposite page 310 in "Report of the Governor of Hawaii," *Annual Reports of the Department of the Interior*, 1901 (Washington, D.C., 1901). One citizen did have a battery-powered car in 1898. See Edward B. Scott, *The Saga of the Sandwich Islands*, Vol. 1 (Lafayette, Ind., 1968), 298.
14. D[uncan] A. Carmichael, "Report of Transactions at Honolulu, H. I. [October 2, 1898 to October 31, 1899]," in *Annual Report of the Supervising Surgeon-General of the Marine-Hospital Service of the United States for the Fiscal Year 1899* (Washington, D.C., 1901), 44; *U.S. House Documents*, 66 (1897), 55th Congress, 2nd Session, No. 483, p. 1248.
15. [C. E. Mann], "Report of Maj. C. E. Mann concerning conditions, sanitary and medical, in Honolulu and the Hawaiian islands," *Report of the Surgeon-General of the Army to the Secretary of War, 1896* (Washington, D.C., 1896), 128–30. On the inspection system, see Robert Barde, "Prelude to Plague: Public Health and Politics at America's Pacific Gateway, 1899," *JHM*, Vol. 58, No. 2 (April 2003), 156.

CHAPTER 2

1. The following brief account of Hawaiian history at the end of the nineteenth century rests upon several previous studies. Among them are Liliuokalani, *Hawaii's Story by Hawaii's Queen* (reprint of 1898 edition; Rutland, Vt., and Tokyo, 1989); Ralph S. Kuykendall and A. Grove Day, *Hawaii: A History* (New York, 1948); Lawrence H. Fuchs, *Hawaii Pono: "Hawaii the Excellent": An Ethnic and Political History* (Honolulu, 1961); Gavan Daws, *Shoal of Time: A History of the Hawaiian Islands* (New York, 1968); Olive Wyndette, *Islands of Destiny: A History of Hawaii* (Rutland, Vt., and Tokyo, 1968); Albertine Loomis, *For Whom Are the Stars?* (Honolulu, 1976); Noel Kent, *Hawaii: Islands Under the Influence* (New York, 1983); Rich Budnick, *Stolen Kingdom: An American Conspiracy* (Honolulu, 1992); Michael Dougherty, *To Steal a Kingdom* (Waimanalo, Hawaii, 1992); Lilikala Kame'eleihiwa, *Native Land and Foreign Desire* (Honolulu, 1992); Michael G. Vann, "Contesting Cultures and Defying Dependency: Migration, Nationalism, and Identity in Late 19th Century Hawaii," *Stanford Humanities Review*, Vol. 5, No. 2 (1997); Haunani-Kay Trask, *From a Native Daughter: Colonialism and Sovereignty in Hawaii* (Honolulu, 1999).

2. On Dole, see also Helena G. Allen, *Sanford Ballard Dole: Hawaii's Only President, 1844–1926* (Glendale, Calif., 1988) and Ethel M. Damon, *Sanford Ballard Dole and His Hawaii, with an Analysis of Justice Dole's Legal Opinions* (Alto, Calif., 1957). On Thurston, see also Lorrin A. Thurston, *Memoirs of the Hawaiian Revolution* (Honolulu, 1936) and Andrew Farrell, ed., *Writings of Lorrin A. Thurston* (Honolulu, 1936).

3. On the "whitening" of the Portuguese, see an editorial in *IND*, January 22, 1900, 4, deploring "the unpardonable ignorance" of those in Honolulu who continued to "talk about 'white' people in contrast to 'Portuguese.'"

4. "Auwe ka Pilikia o ka Lahui [The Crisis of Our People]," *KAA*, January 27, 1900, 2, 7.

5. Albert P. Taylor, "The Impress of Cathay in the Hawaiian Islands," in [Overseas Penman Club], *The Chinese of Hawaii* (Honolulu, 1929), 8; Tin-Yuke Char, *The Sandalwood Mountains: Readings and Stories of the Early Chinese in Hawaii* (Honolulu, 1975), 287.

6. On the rapid economic ascent of the Chinese in Honolulu, which was abundantly evident in the 1890s, see Clarence E. Glick, *Sojourners and Settlers: Chinese Migrants in Hawaii* (Honolulu, 1980), 67–101; Frances Carter, Francis Woo, and Puanani Woo, *Exploring Honolulu's Chinatown* (Honolulu, 1988), 9; Mui King-Chau, "The Chinese as Builders of Hawaii," *Pan-Pacific*, Vol. 1, No. 3 (October–December 1937), in Nancy Foon Young, ed., *Asian-Americans in Hawaii* (Honolulu, 1975), 39.

7. On Ah Leong and Hong Quon, see Chung Kun Ai, *My Seventy-Nine Years in Hawaii* (Hong Kong, 1960), 189–90. On Wong Chow, see [Overseas Penman Club], *The Chinese of Hawaii*, 9.

8. Char, *Sandalwood Mountains*, Appendix G, 288–92; "Voice of the Chinese Colony Declares Itself in a Big Mass Meeting," in Young, 67–70.

9. James G. Y. Ho, "Downtown Historic Anecdotes: Honolulu Chinatown Fires of 1886–1900–1902," *Downtown Planet* (November 4, 2002), 7, 13; telephone conversation with Ho, November 13, 2002. Ho is president and historian of the Hawaiian Chinese Multicultural Museum and Archives in Honolulu and has been collecting oral histories in the city's Chinese community since the 1950s.

10. Lorrin A. Thurston, *A Hand-book on the Annexation of Hawaii* (St. Joseph, Mich., 1897).

11. For an excellent discussion of the congressional debates over how to handle forms of government for the various island territories acquired during this period, see Lanny Thompson, "The Imperial Republic: A Comparison of the Insular Territories under U.S. Dominion after 1898," *Pacific Historical Review*, Vol. 71, No. 4 (November 2002), 535–74.

12. Fifty-fifth Congress, Sess. II, Res. 55, 1898.

CHAPTER 3

1. For a report on the *Nippon Maru* incident in Honolulu, see Carmichael File, MAM.
2. The *Nippon Maru* touched off a public dispute in San Francisco. See Robert Barde, "Prelude to Plague: Public Health and Politics at America's Pacific Gateway, 1899," *JHM*, Vol. 58, No. 2 (April 2003), 153–86; and Marilyn Chase, *The Barbary Plague: The Black Death in Victorian San Francisco* (New York, 2003), 12, 28.
3. *HIN*, 425.
4. For the *Manchuria* rumor, see Li Ling Ai, *Life Is for a Long Time: A Chinese Hawaiian Memoir* (New York, 1972), 169; M. J. Keeling and C. A. Gilligant, "Metapopulation Dynamics of Bubonic Plague," *Nature*, Vol. 407 (2000), 903–6.
5. Gu Jinhui, *Tan Dao Ji Shi* [Historical Record of Hawaii] (Shanghai, 1907 [reprint 1988]), 141. Gu's text used the term *shi zheng* to describe these initial opinions, in contrast to the phrase *wen yu*, implying a more disastrous epidemic, which he subsequently applied to the plague itself; Li, *Life Is for a Long Time*, 170–71. Jerome J. Platt, Maurice E. Jones, and Arleen Kay Platt, *The Whitewash Brigade: The Hong Kong Plague of 1894* (London, 1998), 48. The plant used was probably Isatidis Radix, imported from China.
6. Clarence E. Glick, *Sojourners and Settlers: Chinese Migrants in Hawaii* (Honolulu, 1980), 233.
7. Dole to Baker, July 30, 1895, Dole Papers, HMC.
8. [C. E. Mann], "Report of Maj. C. E. Mann concerning conditions, sanitary and medical, in Honolulu and the Hawaiian islands," *Report of the Surgeon-General of the Army to the Secretary of War, 1896* (Washington, D.C., 1896), 128–30; Frederick L. Hoffman, *The Sanitary Progress and Vital Statistics of Hawaii* (Honolulu, 1915).
9. Dole to Baker, Oct. 17, 1895, Dole Papers, HMC.
10. Glick, *Sojourners and Settlers*, 232–35.
11. Li, *Life Is for a Long Time*, 14.
12. On the Canton Medical School, see Chimin K. Wong and Lien-The Wu, *History of Chinese Medicine* (National Quarantine Service, Shanghai, 1936), passim and 375–76 for the link to German missionary societies.
13. Li, *Life Is for a Long Time*, 19.
14. Li File, MAM.
15. Li, *Life Is for a Long Time*, 1–36, 60–72, 92–96, 100, 133–83, 191–204.
16. Herbert File, MAM.
17. The English-language press reported only that "a Chinese doctor" informed the Board members, but several sources closer to the Chinese situation, including Li's daughter, confirmed that Li was the physician who went to the

Board. See Li, *Life Is for a Long Time*, 168–73; Li File, MAM; *PCA*, December 13, 1899, 1, 9.

18. Li, *Life Is for a Long Time*, 168–73; *KAA*, December 16, 1899, 5.

19. MBH, 102–4.

20. *PCA*, December 13, 1899; "Poha ka Mai Fiva Eleele . . . [Black Fever Erupts]," *KAA*, December 16, 1899, 3.

21. *AHW*, January 20, 1900, 1; *PCA*, December 13, 1899, 1–3.

CHAPTER 4

1. Most of the biographical information that follows is from the Emerson File, MAM. Material from other sources will be cited separately.

2. Minutes of the Board of Health Meetings, July 1, 1868 to June 25, 1881, 180, 182, 186, 211, HSA.

3. I am grateful to Heidi Lyons of the Boston University Alumni Medical Library for information about Peirce's medical education. On Sarah Eliza Peirce Emerson generally, see http://hml.org/mmhc/mdindex/semerson.html, accessed April 4, 2003; [Polk] *Husted's Directory of Honolulu and Hawaiian Territory, 1900/01* (Honolulu, 1901), 54.

4. Olive Wyndette, *Islands of Destiny: A History of Hawaii* (Rutland, Vt., and Tokyo, 1968), 203–4; *FRI*, February 1894, 10.

5. Minutes of the Meetings of the Board of Health, June 25, 1881 to Dec. 31, 1888, 101, HSA; *PCA*, November 21, 1887.

6. Nathaniel Emerson, *The Long Voyages of the Ancient Hawaiians* (Honolulu, 1893). This was an expanded version of a paper he read before the Hawaiian Historical Society on May 18, 1893. In 1903, Emerson translated David Malo's *Moolelo Hawaii* as *Hawaiian Antiquities*, and the Bureau of American Ethnography published Emerson's *Unwritten Literature of Hawaii: Sacred Songs of the Hula* (Washington, D.C., 1909) He wrote many other similar pieces. His papers, which are valued primarily for their Hawaiian-language materials, are now at the Huntington Library.

7. Minutes of the Meetings of the Board of Health, June 25, 1881 to Dec. 31, 1888, 140, HSA.

8. Day File, MAM; "In Memoriam: Francis Root Day, M.D.," a pamphlet in the Frances L. Folsom Papers, Buffalo and Erie County Historical Society Archives, Buffalo, New York.

9. Wood File, MAM.

10. See *Hawaiian Almanac and Annual* (Honolulu), Thomas G. Thrum, compiler, for the years 1897–1900.

11. Carmichael File, MAM; D[uncan]. A. Carmichael, "Report of Transactions at the Port of Honolulu, Territory of Hawaii, During the Fiscal Year ended

June 30, 1900," in *Annual Report of the Supervising Surgeon-General of the Marine-Hospital Service of the United States for the Fiscal Year 1900* (Washington, D.C., 1900), 440–43. On the evolution of the Marine Hospital Service, see Bess Furman, *A Profile of the United States Public Health Service, 1798–1948* (Washington, D.C., 1973), 234; Ralph Chester Williams, *The United States Public Health Service, 1798–1950* (Washington, D.C., 1951), 262–70; and John Parascandola, "Public Health Service," in George Thomas Kurian, editor-in-chief, *A Historical Guide to the U.S. Government* (New York, 1998), 487–93.

12. C. E. Camp to Walter Wyman, October 10, 1899, MHS.
13. Carmichael File, MAM.
14. Hoffman File, MAM.

CHAPTER 5

1. *PCA*, December 13, 1899, 1; December 15, 1899, 4.
2. See, for example, an editorial in *IND*, January 3, 1900, 4, which justified "steady blows" against plague, lest Honolulu end up like Hong Kong, where plague in some form had held on for "the past two hundred years"; *IND*, December 13, 1899, 3.
3. On the fear among nonwhites, see "Aohe Laau Lapaau no ka Hoola Ana i Keia Ano Mai Weliweli [No Medication to Treat This Dreadful Disease]," *KAA*, December 16, 1899, 5; *HGZ*, December 15, 1899, 4; *PCA*, December 15, 1899, 4; *EBU*, December 12, 1899, 4; *IND*, December 13, 1899, 3.
4. *HIN*, 427.
5. MBH, December 12, 1899, 103; D. W. Ketcham, Adjutant, Order No. 270, December 13, 1899; Blair D. Taylor to Surgeon General, December 15, 18, and 22, 1899, MHS.
6. For an excellent discussion of this mind-set, see Mary P. Sutphen, "Not What, but Where: Bubonic Plague and the Reception of Germ Theories in Hong Kong and Calcutta, 1894–1897," *JHM*, Vol. 52, No. 1 (January 1997), 81–113; similar ideas are explored in Susan Craddock, *City of Plagues: Disease, Poverty, and Deviance in San Francisco* (Minneapolis, 2000); *HIN*, 428.
7. Fire had swept the district in 1886, so most of the buildings standing in 1899 were of relatively recent construction. See Clarence E. Glick, *Sojourners and Settlers: Chinese Migrants in Hawaii* (Honolulu, 1980), 12–134.
8. MBH, December 14 and 15, 1899, 107–10; *PCA*, December 14, 1899, 9.
9. For an estimate of ten thousand people, see the remarks of Dr. F. R. Day quoted in a letter to the editor of *PCA*, December 18, 1899, 1; Dion-Margrit Coschigano, "Chinatown: A History of Change," http://www.chinatownhi.com, accessed March 3, 2003.

10. Data on employment and economic status can be found in Glick, *Sojourners and Settlers*, 102–60; and Paul Kimm-Chow Goo, "Building Hawaii's Prosperity," in [Overseas Penman Club], *The Chinese of Hawaii* (Honolulu, 1929), 13; in 1894, the *Hawaiian Star* had estimated the number of vagrants in Chinatown at eight hundred. See Tin-Yuke Char, *The Sandalwood Mountains: Readings and Stories of the Early Chinese in Hawaii* (Honolulu, 1975), Appendix G, 288.

11. Yansheng Ma Lum and Raymond Mun Kong Lum, *Sun Yat-Sen in Hawaii: Activities and Supporters* (Honolulu, 1999).

12. Chung Kun Ai, *My Seventy-Nine Years in Hawaii* (Hong Kong, 1960), 189–91.

13. The thick file of Yang's correspondence with the Board of Health, for example, is overwhelmingly concerned with matters of business and trade. See HBH, Series 334-26; Gu Jinhui [Gu, sometimes Goo, Kim Fui], *Tan Dao Ji Shi* [The Historical Record of Hawaii] (Shanghai, 1907), 148–58.

14. For an example, see *IND*, March 21, 1900, 4; Char, *The Sandalwood Mountains*; Glick, *Sojourners and Settlers*; Li, Ling Ai, *Life Is for a Long Time: A Chinese Hawaiian Memoir* (New York, 1972).

15. Ernest K. Wakukawa, *A History of the Japanese People in Hawaii* (Honolulu, 1938), 84–111; Gary Y. Okihiro, *Cane Fires: The Anti-Japanese Movement in Hawaii, 1865–1945* (Philadelphia, 1991).

16. Morita Sakae, *Hawaii Nihonjin Hatten Shi* [History of Japanese Development in Hawaii] (Waipahu, Hawaii, 1921); Wakukawa, *Japanese People in Hawaii*, 99–123.

17. Soga Yasutaro, *Gojunenkan No Hawaii Kaiko* [My Fifty Years Memoirs in Hawaii] (Osaka, 1953), 82.

18. File from the Japanese consul, HBH, Series 334-26; *YS* advertisements for 1897, which include the prominent Drs. Ogawa, Mori, and Uchida already in practice; licensure letters from the Board of Health to Drs. Soga, Ota, Yanagihara, Haida, and Katsuki, in HBH, Correspondence, Vol. 23, Outgoing letters; Soga, *Gojunenkan No Hawaii Kaiko*, 94.

19. Accurate numbers for Hawaiians in Chinatown are hard to determine. White sources generally offer vague estimates that appear on the low side. The numbers used here are extrapolated from figures in *KAA*, February 3, 1900.

20. Soga, *Gojunenkan No Hawaii Kaiko*, 83.

21. U.S. Bureau of the Census, *Twelfth Census of the United States*, Vol. 1 (Washington, D.C., 1901), 613; for reference to "a Spaniard," see *PCA*, December 27, 1899, 13; for the name and identification of Nakauaila, see *KAA*, December 16, 1899, 2.

22. C[lifford]. B. Wood, "A Brief History Medicine in Hawaii," *Transactions of the First Annual Meeting of the Hawaiian Territorial Medical Association* (Honolulu, 1926), 22. The numbers, and hence the magnitude of the problems he faced, seem to have been inflated a bit as Wood grew older.

23. *AHW*, December 16, 1899, 6; *PCA*, December 16, 1899, 2.

24. *PCA*, December 15, 1899, 14; "Aole no i Loli ae ke Kulana—Eia no ke Pahola mai new; Kapu no Alanui [No Change in Status—Spread Still Seen; Streets Restricted]" *KAA*, December 16, 1899, 2, in which *KAA* announces the suspension of *Ka Makaainana* and the quarantine-induced efforts of *Nupepa Kuokoa* to relocate outside Chinatown and publish on a temporary basis until the quarantine could be lifted; "Oili Hou ka Mai Bubonika [Another Occurrence of the Bubonic Plague]," *KAA*, December 16, 1899, 2; *IND*, December 14, 1899, 4.

25. *PCA*, December 16, 1899, 2; MBH, 108.

26. *EBU*, December 27, 1899, 1.

27. *AHW*, December 6, 1899, 8; Gu, *Tan Dao Ji Shi*, 141–42.

28. "He Hana Pahaohao [Incredible Acts]," *KAA*, December 23, 1899, 5; "Aohe Oiaio oia mau Lono [No Truth to the Reports]," December 23, 1899, 5.

29. *IND*, December 29, 1899, 4, and January 8, 1900, 4; *PCA*, December 13, 1899, 14.

30. Morita, ed., *Hawaii Nihonjin Hatten Shi*, 585; Wood to Saito, April 22, 1900, FO and EX Files, Local Officials, HBH.

31. Jerome J. Platt, Maurice E. Jones, and Arleen Kay Platt, *The Whitewash Brigade: The Hong Kong Plague of 1894* (London, 1998), 71; Charles F. Craig, "The Bubonic Plague from a Sanitary Standpoint," *Pacific Medical Journal*, Vol. 43 (1900), 588.

32. Most European Americans were well aware of the Chinese antipathy to cremation. See Anna Leadingham to unknown, n.d. [ca. December 30, 1899, on the basis of internal evidence], Manuscript Collections, HHS; Platt et al., *The Whitewash Brigade*, 51; *EBU*, December 13, 1899, 1.

33. *PCA*, December 13, 1899, 1; Leadingham to unknown, n.d.; Forrest J. Pinkerton, "Rat Menace Started Public Health Projects," reprint from *Hawaii Magazine*, July 17, 1943, MAM.

CHAPTER 6

1. *PCA*, December 16, 1899, 1; *IND*, December 14, 1899, 4.

2. Technically, McGrew refounded the Hawaiian Medical Society, since a moribund precursor had been established in 1856.

3. John Strayer McGrew File, MAM.

4. *PCA*, December 13, 1899, 3; December 14, 1899, 13.

5. *IND*, December 16, 1899, 4; Henri Goulden McGrew entry, "In Memoriam," at http://hml.org/mmhc/index.html. Henri admitted that he could not recognize the diseases he was supposed to be addressing.

6. For a trenchant editorial on this point, which again sarcastically cites the valiant "little guinea pig," see *IND*, December 18, 1899, 4; *EBU*, December 18, 1899, 1; *IND*, December 18, 1899, 1.

7. *PCA*, December 18, 1899, 13; McGrew File, MAM.
8. [Polk's] *Husted's Directory of Honolulu and Hawaiian Territory, 1900/01* (Honolulu, [1901]), 62; *IND*, December 15, 1899, 4; *PCA*, December 19, 1899, 12.
9. *PCA*, December 14, 1899, 16.
10. *PCA*, December 18, 1899, 4; *EBU*, December 19, 1899, 4; December 20, 1899, 4; *IND*, December 19, 1899, 4; MBH, December 12, 1899, 109; *PCA*, December 16, 1899, 3.
11. "He Hoopalaleha na Ona Waiwai [Land Owners Remain Indifferent]," *KAA*, December 23, 1899, 5.
12. *PCA*, December 18, 1899, 1.
13. *PCA*, December 19, 1899, 1; Sakae Morita, ed., *Hawai Nihonjin Hatten Shi* [History of Japanese Development in Hawaii] (Waipahu, Hawaii, 1921), 587.
14. "Ke Kaikamahine Ma'i Geramania o Iwilei [The Sick German Girl of Iwilei]," *KAA*, December 23, 1899, 5.
15. *PCA*, December 20, 1899, 14.
16. *PCA*, December 23, 1899, 3; Anna Leadingham to unknown, n.d. [ca. December 30, 1899, on the basis of internal evidence], Manuscript Collections, HHS.
17. MBH, December 20, 1899, 112–13; *PCA*, December 21, 1899, 4, 5.
18. See, for example, the editorial comment in *PCA*, December 2, 1899, 4; *IND*, December 22 and 23, 1899; MBH, December 25, 1899, 115.
19. *PCA*, December 26, 1899, 1, 3.
20. *PCA*, December 26, 1899, 3.
21. *IND*, December 27, 1899, 4.
22. *PCA*, December 26, 1899, 3; "Paa ke Kulana . . . [City Under Quarantine . . .]," *KAA*, January 6, 1900, 1.
23. *PCA*, December 27, 1899, 13; MBH, December 25, 1899, 118.
24. MBH, December 25, 1899, 118–19; *PCA*, December 27, 1899, 4.
25. *IND*, December 27, 1899, 4; *PCA*, December 27, 1899, 13.
26. Li File, MAM; *IND*, December 29, 1899, 4.
27. *PCA*, December 28, 1899, 13.
28. Gu Jinhui, *Tan Dao Ji Shi* [Historical Record of Hawaii] (Shanghai, 1907 [reprint 1988]), 142.
29. Mitamura File, MAM; *EBU*, December 28, 1899, 1; *PCA*, December 28, 1899, 13; *HGZ*, December 15, 1899, 4.
30. *PCA*, December 28, 1899, 13.
31. "Pioo ke Kulanakauhale—Paa Hou no Alanui i ke Kiai ia e no Koa—Hookapu ia na Poe o ka Apna e Hoomalu Mua ia Aole e Puke Iwaho—Eia no ka Ma'i ke Pahola mai nei [City in Panic—The Streets Once Again Closed and Guarded by Troops—People within the Quarantined Area Restricted from Leaving—The Disease Spreads]," *KAA*, December 30, 1899, 3.
32. *EBU*, December 28, 1899, 1; December 30, 1899, 1.
33. *EBU*, December 28, 1899, 1; *PCA*, December 29, 1899, 5.

CHAPTER 7

1. *PCA*, December 30, 1899, 9.
2. MBH, December 25, 1899, 120.
3. *FRI*, Vol. 58, No. 1 (January 1900), 3.
4. These and subsequent quotes, unless separately noted, are taken from a detailed discussion of this meeting that appeared in *PCA*, January 1, 1900, 19.
5. The piece Thurston had read was almost certainly A. Shadwell, "The Plague in Oporto," *The Nineteenth Century*, Vol. XLVI (July–December 1899), 833–47.
6. *EBU*, January 1, 1900, 1.
7. MBH, December 30, 1899, 121.
8. *PCA*, January 1, 1900, 19.
9. Many letters addressed to the Marine Hospital Service in Washington attested to the continued debate over the efficacy of various vaccines and prophylactic serums. See Correspondence, Box 645, MHS; *PCA*, January 31, 1900; Radhika Ramasubban, "Imperial Health in British India, 1857–1900," in Roy Macleod and Milton Lewis, eds., *Disease, Medicine, and Empire: Perspectives on Western Medicine and the Experience of European Expansion* (London and New York, 1988), 54–55; United States Public Health Service scrapbooks, "Bubonic Plague, No. 1," 75, PHS; Alfred Harburld [?], Special Agent of the Government of Hawaii, to Surgeon General Walter Wyman, January 21, 1900, with endorsements from Wyman's staff; and Major Blair D. Taylor, Surgeon, U.S. Army, to Reypren, February 1, 1900; both in Correspondence Files, Box 645, MHS.
10. On this point in general, see "Discussion of Calvert and Kinyoun on Plague," *Journal of the American Medical Association*, Vol. 42 (1904), 238–39, in which speakers point out how much more the medical profession knew about plague in 1904 "than it did even two or three years ago."
11. Honolulu Board of Health to the Board of Health of New South Wales, January 31, 1900, Outgoing Correspondence, Vol. 23, HBH, discusses some of the early disinfection experiments with sulfuric acid and formalin; "The Plague: Action of Gaseous Disinfectants on the Plague Bacillus," *British Medical Journal* (1899), 433–34; E. Klein, "Experiments on Disinfection of Bacillus Pestis with 'Cyllin,' 'Absolute Phenol,' and 'Formalin,'" *Public Health* (London), Vol. 16 (1903–04), 563–66.
12. *PCA*, January 1, 1900, 19.
13. MBH, December 30, 1899, 121–22.
14. *PCA*, December 30, 1899, 4; January 1, 1900, 19.
15. Jerome Platt, Maurice Jones, and Arleen Platt, *The Whitewash Brigade: The Hong Kong Plague of 1894* (London, 1998), 77–78.
16. *FRI*, Vol. 58, No. 1 (January 1900), 3.
17. Honolulu Board of Health to the Board of Health of New South Wales, Jan. 31, 1900, Outgoing Correspondence, Vol. 23, HBH; MBH, March 3, 1900,

318; *PCA*, May 17, 1900; Herbert P. Williams, "Honolulu's Contention with the Plague," *Sanitarian* (1900), 327. The effort to find alternative disinfectants continued for many years. See, for example, Blair D. Taylor to Surgeon General, December 29, 1899, and Edward Browaert, Consul-General of France in New York City, to Surgeon General, January 13, 1902, both in Box 645, MHS.

18. MBH, December 31, 1900, 124.

19. *FRI*, Vol. 58, No. 1 (January 1900), 3; MBH, January 2, 1900, 127.

20. *PCA*, January 1, 1900, 14, January 2, 1900, 4; *FRI*, Vol. 58, No. 1 (January 1900), 3.

21. *HGZ*, January 5, 1900, 4; "Is the City Quarantined?" *AHW*, January 20, 1900, 4; *EBU*, January 1, 1900, 4; January 2, 1900, 3, 4; January 4, 1900, 1; *IND*, January 3 and 5, 1900.

22. Bishop Estate to the Board of Health, January 9, 1900, and February 2, 1900; Achi and Johnson, attorneys for Hawaii Land Company, Limited, to Board of Health, January 18, 1900; Jas. McLean, agent for Mrs. M. A. Gray ["who resides in San Francisco"] to the Board of Health, January 18, 1900, in "Incoming Letters: 1900, Fire Protests," Series 334-27, HBH; Report of "Mr. Bolte for the Silvera estate" in MBH, January 5, 1900, 128; Cecil Brown, attorney for John Ena, lessee of the property of L. L. McCandless, to the Board of Health, January 18, 1900, in "Incoming Letters: 1900, Fire Protests," Series 334-27, HBH.

23. Enoch Johnson to the Board of Health, January 11, 1900; Achi and Johnson, attorneys for Hawaii Land Company, Limited, to the Board of Health, January 18, 1900; W. W. Ahana to the Board of Health, January 12, 1900; attorneys for A. V. Gear and Fred Harrison to the Board of Health, January 13, 1900; and Charles H. Rose to the Board of Health, January 18, 1900, all in "Incoming Letters: 1900, Fire Protests," Series 334-27, HBH.

24. Mitamura File, MAM; "Hooweliweli ia na Kauka Iapana [Japanese Doctors Threatened]," *KAA*, January 13, 1900, 1; *EBU*, January 15, 1900, 1, January 8, 1900, 1; protest from the residents of block 4 to the Board of Health, January 15, 1900, in "Incoming Letters: 1900, Fire Protests," Series 334-27, HBH.

25. Exhibit F, File for Japanese consul Saito, "Incoming Correspondence," Series 334–26, HBH.

26. *IND*, January 13, 1900, 4; January 11, 1900, 4; "Laweia no ka Homalu ana [Taken Under Quarantine]," *KAA*, January 6, 1900, 1.

27. *HGZ*, January 5, 1900, 3; *IND*, January 13, 1900, 4. In Thos. G. Thrum, compiler, *Hawaiian Almanac and Annual for 1901* (Honolulu, 1900), 99, is a reference to "not a few concealed cases of sickness" occurring among Hawaiians. But that is the only such reference I came across, and the Board of Health never alleged any such cover-ups or lack of cooperation among Hawaiians. See also the entry for January 29, 1900, in "Outgoing Letters," Vol. 23, HBH; *KAA*, January 13, 1900, 2.

28. *EBU*, January 2, 1900, 1; *Tan Shang Xin Bao Long Ji* [Hawaiian Chinese News], January 5, 1900; Yang Wei Pin to the Board of Health, January 2, 1900, "Incoming Correspondence," Series 334-26, HBH.
29. See C. Q. Yee Hop, Pang Chong, Pang See, and Ehun Yong to the Board of Health, January 18, 1900, in "Incoming Letters: 1900, Fire Protests," Series 334-27, HBH. The files contain many other letters of a similar nature from Chinese property owners.
30. Petition from block 7, January 15, 1900, in "Incoming Correspondence," Series 334-26, HBH.
31. MBH, January 1, 1900, 125–26.

CHAPTER 8

1. MBH, January 4, 1900, 130.
2. MBH, January 3, 1900, 129.
3. N. B. Emerson to "Sister Dora and Bro. Joe," January 4, 1900, Emerson Papers, HUN.
4. MBH, January 3, 1900, 128–29; *FRI*, Vol. 558, No. 2 (February 1900) later reported the amount drawn as $270,000.
5. *HGZ*, January 9, 1900, 7; *PCA*, January 4, 1900, 5; *EBU*, January 3, 1900, 1. The change of Board presidents had been cleared in advance with the Dole administration, which also agreed to urge the United States to incorporate an independent Board of Health into "the form of government to be adopted for the Hawaiian Islands."
6. MBH, January 5, 1900, 131.
7. *EBU*, December 13, 1899, 1.
8. MBH, January 5, 1900, 132–33.
9. *PCA*, December 3, 1899, 3.
10. *HGZ*, January 9, 1900, 1; *EBU*, January 8, 1900, 6.
11. *PCA*, January 8, 1900, 1, 3. *HGZ*, January 9, 1900, 1; *EBU*, January 8, 1900, 6.
12. *IND*, January 8, 1900, 4.
13. *PCA*, January 8, 1900, 1; *HGZ*, January 9, 1900, 6.
14. *EBU*, January 8, 1900, 1.
15. *HGZ*, January 9, 1900, 6.
16. *PCA*, January 9, 1900, 4.
17. *PCA*, January 9, 1900, 4.
18. *HGZ*, January 9, 1900, 4; *PCA*, January 10, 1900, 2.
19. See John F. Colburn to the *Advertiser*, reprinted in *HGZ*, January 12, 1900, 2.
20. *PCA*, January 11, 1900, 3.
21. *PCA*, January 13, 1900, 14.
22. *HGZ*, January 9, 1900, 1; *PCA*, January 11, 1900, 7.
23. *IND*, January 11, 1900, 4.

24. MBH, January 7, 1900, 136, January 10, 1900, 145; Honolulu Board of Health to Alexander Young, January 12, 1900, Correspondence, Outgoing Letters, Vol. 23, HBH. For the number of carpenters, see Honolulu Board of Health to Board of Health, Sydney, New South Wales, January 31, 1900, in Vol. 23, Correspondence, Outgoing Letters, HBH.

25. MBH, January 7–10, 1900, 136–63; Honolulu Board of Health to Board of Health of Sydney, New South Wales; MBH, January 8, 1900, 144; *PCA*, January 13, 1900, 1.

CHAPTER 9

1. "Lawelawe Oolea o Kauai [Strict Orders on Kauai]," *KAA*, January 6, 1900, 2; *PCA*, January 15, 1900, 3, January 17, 1900, 4, and related stories that week.

2. *IND*, January 11, 1900, 1; MBH, January 7, 1900, 136, January 10, 1900, 160, and passim; *PCA*, January 12, 1900, 9, January 17, 1900, 4.

3. Journal of N. B. Emerson, entry for January 28, 1900, HUN. This problem proved troubling and ongoing. See *IND*, February 15, 1900, 4.

4. *IND*, January 9, 1900, 4.

5. See C. B. Wood to Dole, January 9, 1900, HBH.

6. For an example, see *IND*, March 3, 1900, 4.

7. Exhibit F, File of the Japanese Consul, Incoming Correspondence, Series 334-26, HBH.

8. "Na Hana Kikua Hou a ka Ahahui Kokua Manawalea Hawaii [Other acts of the Aid by the Hawaiian Relief Services Association]," "Ka Hui Kikua Manawalea Hawaii [Hawaiian Relief Services Association]," *KAA*, January 20, 1900, 3.

9. See, for example, letters to the Hawaiian Relief Society, the Chinese consul, and the Japanese consul on February 8, 1900, authorizing money for relief efforts, in Outgoing Correspondence, Vol. 23, HBH; *KAA*, January 20, 1900, 3, also expressed gratitude to the Board, because they "heeded the pleas of the Association."

10. *HGZ*, January 9, 1900, 2, January 27, 1900, 4; *EBU*, January 10, 1900, 1, January 15, 1900, 1, January 17, 3, 6.

11. J. P. Cooke to Dole, January 11, 1900, HBH.

12. "He Ku Maoli i ka Walohia [Sadly . . .]," *KAA*, January 6, 1900, 4; "Na Make o ke Kulanakauhale nei [Death Toll in the City]," January 6, 1900, p. 7.

13. See, for example, George Manson to W. W. Carter, Esq., complaining about a Portuguese named Domingos Ferreira, who was caught breaking and entering in the name of the Board of Health. Incoming Correspondence, Series 334-26, HBH; *IND*, January 13, 1900, 4; *EBU*, January 18, 1900, 4.

14. *EBU*, January 15, 1900, 1.

15. "He Oiaio Anei hoi Keia? [Is This True?]," *KAA*, January 20, 1900, 2.
16. *EBU*, January 15, 1900, 1; Soga Yasutaro, *Gojunenkan No Hawaii Kaiko* [My Fifty Years Memoirs in Hawaii] (Honolulu, 1954), 82; Sakae Morita, ed., *Hawai Nihonjin Hatten Shi* [The History of Japanese Development in Hawaii] (Waipahu, Hawaii, 1921), 594.
17. Saito to C. B. Wood, January 17, 1900, HBH.
18. C. B. Wood to Saito, January 17, 1900, HBH; *IND*, January 19, 1900, 4.
19. *PCA*, January 13, 1900, 5.
20. For the most recent example, see *Hawaiian Almanac and Annual for 1900* (Honolulu, 1900), 171. Previous *Almanac*s regularly chronicled accidental fires in the area. For an excellent account of the largest of those earlier accidental fires, see Richard A. Greer, "'Sweet and Clean': the Chinatown Fire of 1886," *HJH*, Vol. 10 (1976), 33–51.
21. *PCA*, January 2, 1900, 9.
22. *PCA*, January 13, 1900, 1; *FRI*, Vol. 58, No. 2 (February 1900), 3; *EBU*, January 4, 1900, 4.
23. *PCA*, January 13, 1900, 14, January 11, 1900, 4.
24. *PCA*, January 11, 1900, 2, 5; *KAA*, January 13, 1900, 1, January 20, 1900, 1.
25. *IND*, January 16, 17, 1900, 4; *FRI*, Vol. 58, No. 2 (February 1900), 4; *EBU*, January 14, 15, 16, 1900.
26. *EBU*, January 20, 1900, 1.
27. *PCA*, January 14, 1900, 3, January 16, 1900, 1; MBH, January 17, 1900, 181.
28. *PCA*, January 16, 1900, 1, January 20, 1900, 9.
29. *PCA*, January 13, 1900, 1, January 17, 1900, 7; *KAA*, January 20, 1900, 7; *EBU*, December 13, 1899, 1, December 14, 1899, 4.
30. *PCA*, January 15, 1900, 4; January 16, 1900, 4; January 19, 1900, 4.
31. *PCA*, January 16, 1900, 4.
32. MBH, January 15–19, 1900, 173–86; Chung Kun Ai, *My Seventy-Nine Years in Hawaii* (Hong Kong, 1960), 192.
33. *PCA*, January 20, 1900, 1, 9.

CHAPTER 10

1. *PCA*, January 17, 1900, 1.
2. Richard A. Greer, "'Sweet and Clean': The Chinatown Fire of 1886," *HJH*, Vol. 10 (1976), 35.
3. All of Honolulu's newspapers carried extensive coverage of the fire after the fact. The account that follows is put together from those stories collectively. Only direct quotations will be noted separately.
4. Frank Davey, "Through Plague and Fire in Honolulu, Hawaiian Islands," undated typescript memoir, 4, Ms Doc 108, BMA.
5. Davey, "Through Plague and Fire"; *Honolulu Star-Bulletin*, April 21, 2001.

6. *PCA,* January 22, 1900, 2; "Detailed Record of the Second Fire of Chinatown [in Chinese]," in [Overseas Penman Club], *The Chinese of Hawaii* (Honolulu, 1929), 42.
7. *EBU,* January 20, 1900, 1.
8. Chung Kun Ai, *My Seventy-Nine Years in Hawaii* (Hong Kong, 1960), 193.
9. *EBU,* January 20, 1900, 1; Soga Yasutaro, *Gojunenkan No Hawaii Kaiko* [My Fifty Years Memoirs in Hawaii] (Honolulu, 1954), 83.
10. *PCA,* January 22, 1900, 3; *EBU,* January 20, 1900, 1; Davey, "Through Plague and Fire," 6 (emphasis in original).
11. *IND,* January 19, 1900, 4; *PCA,* January 22, 1900, 3; January 24, 1900, 10.
12. For the memories of a woman who watched the event from this vantage point when she was a girl, see Helen P. Hoyt, *Aloha, Susan!* (Garden City, N.J., 1961), 75–82.
13. Soga, *Gojunenkan No Hawaii Kaiko,* 83.
14. Davey, "Through Plague and Fire," 6.
15. *PCA,* January 22, 1900, 1.
16. Li Ling Ai, *Life Is for a Long Time: A Chinese Hawaiian Memoir* (New York, 1972), 174.
17. *PCA,* January 22, 1900, 2, 6; *EBU,* January 20, 1900, 1.
18. *PCA,* January 22, 1900, 3; *HIN,* 191–93.
19. *PCA,* January 22, 1900, 3, 6.
20. Gu Jinhui, *Tan Dao Ji Shi* [Historical Record of Hawaii] (Shanghai, 1907 [reprint 1988]), 145.
21. *PCA,* January 24, 1900, 10; petition of Wong Chow, Chun Wing, and others to the Senate investigating committee in *HIN,* 191–93.
22. MBH, January 20, 1900, 189.
23. *FRI,* Vol. 58, No. 2 (February 1900), 3; Davey, "Through Plague and Fire," 7; *EBU,* January 20, 1900, 1.
24. Soga, *Gojunenkan No Hawaii Kaiko,* 83; Davey, "Through Plague and Fire," 6; *PCA,* January 22, 1900, 6.
25. Scrapbook of Mary Sophronia Whitney, 104–17, HHS.
26. *FRI,* Vol. 58, No. 2 (February 1900), 3; Blair D. Taylor to Surgeon General, January 22, 1900, Correspondence Files, MHS.
27. *EBU,* January 21, 1900, 1; *PCA,* January 22, 1900, 3.
28. *PCA,* January 22, 1900, 4.

CHAPTER 11

1. *PCA,* January 22, 1900, 4; *KAA,* January 13, 1900, 2, and January 20, 1900, 2; Richard A. Greer, "'Sweet and Clean': The Chinatown Fire of 1886," *HJH,* Vol. 10 (1976), 40.
2. *FRI,* Vol. 58, No. 2 (February 1900), 5.

3. *EBU*, January 21, 1900, 1.
4. *PCA*, January 22, 1900, 10; *EBU*, January 21, 1900, 1.
5. *EBU*, January 21, 1900, 1; *PCA*, January 22, 1900, 10.
6. MBH, January 22, 1900, 190–93; *FRI*, Vol. 58, No. 2 (February 1900), 4; *IND*, February 26, 1900, 4.
7. *FRI*, Vol. 58, No. 2 (February 1900), 3–4.
8. *EBU*, January 21, 1.
9. *PCA*, January 22, 1900, 7. For a typical example of the Board's having to deal with such problems, see MBH, February 12, 1900, 248–51.
10. MBH, January 22, 1900, 193; *IND*, February 12, 1900, 4.
11. For a fine summary of these efforts, see Lana Iwamoto, "The Plague and Fire of 1899–1900 in Honolulu," *Hawaiian Historical Review*, Vol. 2 (1967), 389–90; *EBU*, February 7, 1900, 1; *IND*, March 9, 1900, 4.
12. *PCA*, January 22, 1900, 4; D[uncan]. A. Carmichael, "Report of Transactions at the Port of Honolulu, Territory of Hawaii, During the Fiscal Year ended June 30, 1900," in *Annual Report of the Supervising Surgeon-General of the Marine-Hospital Service of the United States for the Fiscal Year 1900* (Washington, D.C., 1900), 441.
13. Wong Chow to editor, January 23, 1900, in *PCA*, January 25, 1900, 3. The paper hinted that the letter may have been written by a white man and merely signed by Wong Chow, but concluded that it probably represented Chinese points of view.
14. MBH, January 27, 1900, 211; *EBU*, January 30, 1900, 3.
15. Yang Wei Pin to E. A. Mott [Hawaiian Minister of Foreign Affairs], January 15, 1900, Incoming Correspondence, Series 334-26, HBH; M. C. Amana to Editor, January 20, 1900, reprinted in *PCA*, January 22, 1900, 6, and elsewhere; *PCA*, January 24, 1900, 4.
16. *EBU*, February 2, 1900, 2.
17. Li Ling Ai, *Life Is for a Long Time: A Chinese Hawaiian Memoir* (New York, 1972), 175; MBH, February 8, 1900, 242, February 14, 1900, 266; Gu Jinhui, *Tan Dao Ji Shi* [Historical Record of Hawaii] (Shanghai, 1907 [reprint 1988]), 148–49.
18. *IND*, January 29, 1900, 4.
19. *PCA*, February 5, 1900, 1; Clarence E. Glick, *Sojourners and Settlers: Chinese Migrants in Hawaii* (Honolulu, 1980), 230.
20. *EBU*, March 30, 1900, 1; April 13, 1900, 4; *PCA*, January 24, 1900, 6; January 25, 1900, 4.
21. Li, *Life Is for a Long Time*, 170–71, 174–75.
22. Li, *Life Is for a Long Time*, 177, 178.
23. Telephone interview with James G. Y. Ho, director of the Hawaiian Chinese Multicultural Museum and Archives, November 11, 2002. Ho spent many years gathering oral histories among Honolulu's Chinese residents.

24. See, for example, "Exhibit F" in the separate file of materials from Saito, Incoming Correspondence, Series 334-26, HBH; *EBU*, February 7, 1900, 1; *KAA*, January 27, 1900, 3, 4.

25. Kawata Minoru, ed., *Imin Taiken Ki* [A Chronicle of Immigrant Experience], Vol. 1 (Hiroshima, 1974), 9–10; Frank Davey, "Through Plague and Fire in Honolulu, Hawaiian Islands," undated typescript memoir, 8; Ms Doc 108, BMA; *IND*, January 27, 1900, 4.

26. *PCA*, January 31, 1900, 5; *HGZ*, January 30, 1900, 1, 5; MBH, February 16, 1900, 272; *EBU*, January 30, 1, February 10, 1900, 1.

27. Soga Yasutaro, *Gojunenkan No Hawaii Kaiko* [My Fifty Years Memoirs in Hawaii] (Honolulu, 1954), 84.

28. See, for example, the letter of January 29, 1900, in Outgoing Correspondence, Vol. 23, HBH.

29. *KAA*, January 27, 1900, 4.

30. "Ka Hui Kikua Manawalea Hawaii [Hawaiian Relief Services Association]," *KAA*, January 20, 1900, 3. For commentary on the flap that arose over where to hold Boardman, see *IND*, January 18, 1900, 4.

31. For Hawaiian protests against that policy, see "Na Hana Kapakahi a ke Aupuni—Hoolilo ia ka Hotele Queen i Wahi Hoomalu no na Haole [Mishandling of the Government—Queen Hotel Converted to a Quarantine Facility for Whites]," *KAA*, January 20, 1900, 5.

32. *PCA*, February 5, 1900, 5; February 12, 1900, 10.

CHAPTER 12

1. MBH, January 24, 1900, 196–97; *PCA*, January 25, 1900, 12; January 26, 1900, 9.

2. MBH, January 24, 198–99; "Ke Oili Liilii Nei No—Elua Make a me Hookahi Mai [Cases Spreading—Two Deaths One is Sick]," *KAA*, January 27, 1900, 2.

3. MBH, January 25, 1900, 199; *KAA*, January 27, 1900, 7.

4. Dion-Margrit Coschigano, "Chinatown: A History of Change," http://www.chinatownhi.com (accessed March 3, 2003), estimates that there were 81 Chinese stores outside Chinatown and 72 Chinese stores inside Chinatown in 1896; *PCA*, January 24, 1900, 4; January 27, 1900, 1–2; March 7, 1900, 9.

5. *PCA*, February 6, 1900, 10.

6. *IND*, January 29, 1900, 4; *PCA*, January 29, 1900, 1.

7. *PCA*, January 23, 1900, 5.

8. Sloggett File, MAM.

9. Nathaniel B. Emerson to "Sister Dora and Bro. Joe," January 4, 1900, emphasis in original; Diary of Nathaniel B. Emerson, entry for January 24, 1900, both in HUN.

10. Carmichael File, MAM.

11. *PCA*, January 22, 1900, 9; Emerson Diary, entry for January 24, 1900.
12. *PCA*, January 26, 1900, 1; MBH, February 14, 1900, 265.
13. *PCA*, January 30, 1900, 1, 4; February 1, 1900, 9; February 2, 1900, 2.
14. Honolulu Board of Health to Board of Health, Sydney, New South Wales, January 31, 1900, Vol. 23, Correspondence, Outgoing Letters, HBH.
15. Dole referred to Hoffman's ongoing efforts in the wake of the great fire. See *PCA*, January 22, 1900, 10. Though historians can now recount in some detail the story of British experiments with Haffkine's serum, Hoffman and his colleagues knew only what they could learn from United States consular dispatches relayed to them by the United States Marine Hospital Service. See the report of William T. Fee, U.S. consul in Bombay, September 7, 1899, reprinted in *PCA*, January 31, 1900, 1.
16. Angus Smedley, "Autobiography of an LDS Missionary to Hawaii, 1900–1904," 67–69, Doc. 216, BMA.
17. On the call for vaccines, see also Wilcox (secretary to the Board of Health) to Saito, March 3, 1900, HBH; and Taylor to Reypren, February 1, 1900, Correspondence, Box 645, MHS.
18. Hoffman File, MAM; *PCA*, January 16, 1900, 10; February 2, 1900, 10.
19. *FRI*, Vol. 58, No. 2 (February 1900), 1.
20. See *PCA*, February 3, 1900, 1; February 7, 1900, 5. Robertson boasted that he was king of the rat killers, having dispatched seventeen in his own store. He had also casually handled the bodies of about twenty other dead rats—without taking any special precautions—while helping fellow workers dispose of them.
21. *PCA*, February 3, 1900, 2.
22. "Bubonic Plague No. 1," 196, 199, 201–2, 206, 209, 217. Public Health Service Scrapbooks, PHS.
23. *PCA*, February 5, 1900, 4.
24. *PCA*, February 5, 1900, 1–2, 4.
25. For information about Honolulu's principal stables, see Edward B. Scott, *The Saga of the Sandwich Islands*, Vol. 1 (Lafayette, Ind., 1968), 263; *PCA*, February 6, 1900, 4; February 7, 1900, 2.
26. MBH, February 6, 1900, 233–37, February 9, 1900, 244; *PCA*, February 5, 1900, 1; February 7, 1900, 4; February 9, 1900, 4; February 10, 1900, 7; February 12, 1900, 4; Uldrick Thompson Sr., "Reminiscences of Old Hawaii," 135, typescript in HHS.
27. *PCA*, February 5, 1900, 4, 11; *IND*, January 30, 1900, 4.
28. *PCA*, February 7, 1900, 4; *EBU*, February 7, 1900, 4.
29. MBH, February 2, 1900, 223–27; February 3, 1900, 227–29; *EBU*, February 15, 1900, 1; February 18, 1900, 2.
30. "Bubonic Plague, No. 1," 232, PHS; *EBU*, February 12, 1900; *Tan Shang Xi Bao Long Ji* [Hawaiian Chinese News] (Honolulu), February 9, 1900; *IND*,

February 24, 1900, 4; March 3, 1900, 4; Gu Jinhui, *Tan Dao Ji Shi* [Historical Record of Hawaii] (Shanghai, 1907 [reprint 1988]), 149–52.

31. "Bubonic Plague No. 2," 1, PHS; *PCA*, February 9, 1900, 3; March 7, 1900, 10; March 8, 1900, 5; *KAA*, January 27, 1900, 1, 2; *EBU*, February 7, 1900, 1, 4; February 18, 1900, 2; March 8, 1900, 1.

32. *KAA*, January 27, 1900, 2; *HIN*, 127.

33. *IND*, February 22, 1900, 4.

34. MBH, February 1, 1900, 217–22; *PCA*, February 12, 1900, 3; February 13, 1900, 3.

35. *PCA*, February 12. 1900, 11; February 13, 1900, 3.

36. Gulstan, Bishop of Panopolis, to the Damien Institute, February 12, 1900, HMC.

CHAPTER 13

1. For the continued isolationism on Hawaii, see Dr. Moore to Board of Health, April 10, 1900, in Bubonic Plague File, MAM; for reports from Maui, see Sabey File and Weddick File, MAM; *EBU*, December 12, 1899.

2. W[illiam] H. Chickering to Walter Wyman, March 20, 1900, Correspondence, Box 645, MHS; MBH, February 13, 1900, 252–59; Weddick File, MAM. Weddick, who headed the Kahului physicians' committee, was subsequently presented with a gold watch by the people of Maui for his selfless services during the plague crisis there. Quotes regarding Maui are from *EBU*, February 12, 1900, 1, 4; February 13, 1900, 1; February 15, 1900, 1, 8; and *PCA*, February 13, 1900, 5. The complete Maui story and subsequent reports can be followed in any of the Honolulu papers.

3. *PCA*, February 13, 1900, 10; February 15–19, 1900, passim; MBH, February 14, 1900, 264.

4. Forrest J. Pinkerton, "Rat Menace Started Public Health Projects," reprint from *Hawaii Magazine*, July 17, 1943, MAM; *PCA*, February 14, 1900, 2; MBH, February 13, 1900, 261, March 6, 1900, 327; *PCA*, February 15, 1900, 6; February 16, 1900, 7.

5. MBH, February 19, 1900, 279; *PCA*, February 20, 1900, 7.

6. *PCA*, February 23, 1900, 8.

7. *PCA*, February 24, 1900, 1; *EBU*, February 26, 1900, 1; *IND*, February 23, 1900, 4; Maj. [Oscar F.] Long to Quartermaster General, February 24, 1900, Correspondence, Box No. 645, MHS.

8. For this debate generally, see *PCA*, February 22–27, 1900.

9. MBH, March 1, 1900, 312; *EBU*, February 20, 1900, 4.

10. MBH, February 28, 1900, 308.

11. *IND*, March 2, 1900, 4; March 3, 1900, 5; March 6, 1900, 4; MBH, March 5, 1900, 324.

12. An earlier Natural History and Microscopic Society of amateurs had gone defunct by the mid-1880s, and this new society, as the authority on microscopy in Honolulu has noted, "was a new breed of men, with a different purpose in mind . . . physicians and 'paramedical personnel' . . . members of a generation who were acquainted with the new doctrines and techniques of micro-biology, pathology, and epidemiology. They met not as dilettantes but as scientists, to share their reading and their experiences, in the hope of improving diagnostic procedures in the clinical medicine and public health." O. A. Bushnell, "Much Ado About Little Things: Microscopes and Microscopists," *HJH*, Vol. 3 (1969), 101–10.

13. *PCA*, March 5, 1900, 10.

14. *PCA*, February 8, 1900, 4.

15. *EBU*, March 6, 1900, 1.

16. *PCA*, March 14, 1900, 3.

17. *EBU*, March 13, 1900, 1; *PCA*, March 14, 1900, 3.

18. *PCA*, March 16, 1900, 4; Hoffman File, MAM.

19. *IND*, April 6, 1900, 4; *PCA*, March 30, 1900, 3. Some Japanese apparently used inoculation certificates more than once and for more than one person.

20. See Mori File, MAM; *YS*, 1898–99, passim, and December 23, 1899. I am indebted to Professor Andrew Goble of the University of Oregon for translation of the medical advertisements.

21. See "Reply to 'Helper' by a Layman," *PCA*, April 2, 1900, 10, 15; April 27, 3; *EBU*, March 21, 1900, 1.

22. *PCA*, March 2, 1900, 1, 3; MBH, March 2, 1900, 314.

23. *IND*, March 13, 1900, 4; *PCA*, April 16, 1900, 11; April 26, 1900, 7.

24. *PCA*, March 7, 1900, 5.

25. *PCA*, March 6, 1900, 6; March 7, 9; MBH, March 6, 326.

26. *PCA*, March 9, 1900, 4; March 26, 1900, 6, 14; March 27, 1900, 13.

27. *PCA*, March 31, 1900, 4; April 2, 1900, 15; April 3, 1900, 9.

28. Claims Submitted; 1900 Fire Losses, Records of the Claims Commission, HSA.

29. *HGZ*, February 27, 1900, 1.

30. *PCA*, April 2–9, 1900; *EBU*, March 3, 1900, 1; March 5, 1900, 1.

31. Soga Yasutaro, *Gojunenkan No Hawaii Kaiko* [My Fifty Years Memoirs in Hawaii] (Honolulu, 1954), 85.

32. Soga, *Gojunenkan No Hawaii Kaiko*, 86.

33. *PCA*, April 9, 1900, 6; Soga, *Gojunenkan No Hawaii Kaiko*, 86.

34. *PCA*, April 10, 1900, 10; Soga, *Gojunenkan No Hawaii Kaiko*, 87.

35. *EBU*, April 7, 1900, 4.

36. *PCA*, April 13, 1900, 5; April 19, 1900, 3; *IND*, March 15, 1900, 4.

37. *EBU*, April 13, 17, and 27, 1900, 1; *PCA*, April 13 and 20, 1900, 10; April 18, 1900, 9.

38. For earlier jabs of a similar nature, see *IND*, February 27, 1900, 4.
39. *PCA*, April 19, 1900, 3, May 17, 1900; *EBU*, April 17, 1900, 1.
40. *PCA*, April 20, 1900, 4.
41. *PCA*, April 24, 1900, 3; *IND*, April 11, 1900, 4.
42. *PCA*, April 20, 1900, 9.
43. *PCA*, April 21, 1900, 10, 12.
44. Jobe File, MAM; *PCA*, April 28, 1900, 1; April 30, 1900, 1.

CHAPTER 14

1. U.S. Statutes at Large, 31 (April 30, 1900), 141.
2. *New York Times*, March 2, 1900, 5; Lanny Thompson, "The Imperial Republic: A Comparison of the Insular Territories under U.S. Dominion after 1898," *Pacific Historical Review*, Vol. 71, No. 4 (November 2002), 535–74.
3. "Payment of Judgments on Claims Growing out of Suppression of Bubonic Plague in Hawaii," 57th Congress, *House Reports*, No. 3098.
4. *HIN*, 420–22, and Part 3. The commissioners maintained that they took each claim on its face and made good-faith estimates. But testimony before a special Senate committee makes clear that their procedures had the practical effect of across-the-board discounting.
5. "Records of the Fire Claims Commission, 1901–1903," HSA.
6. Soga Yasutaro, *Gojunenkan No Hawaii Kaiko* [My Fifty Years Memoirs in Hawaii] (Honolulu, 1954), 85–92; *Tanshan Xin Zhongguo Bao* [Hawaiian New China Paper] (Honolulu), n.d.. "The Japanese consul in Hawaii frequently asked the government for the indemnification. . . . The Japanese consul loves his people as his children" and so forth.
7. Gu Jinhui, *Tan Dao Ji Shi* [Historical Record of Hawaii] (Shanghai, 1907 [reprint 1988]), 155–58; *Tanshan Longji Xin Bao* [Hawaiian Chinese News] (Honolulu), February 17, 1900.
8. Clarence E. Glick, *Sojourners and Settlers: Chinese Migrants in Hawaii* (Honolulu, 1980), 381, note 51; Li Ling Ai, *Life Is for a Long Time: A Chinese Hawaiian Memoir* (New York, 1972), 174.
9. Chung Kun Ai, *My Seventy-Nine Years in Hawaii* (Hong Kong, 1960), 192–97.
10. *HIN*, 192.
11. "Business of Chinese Immigrants [in Chinese]," in [Overseas Penman Club], *The Chinese of Hawaii* (Honolulu, 1929), 42; Tin-Yuke Char, ed., *The Sandalwood Mountains: Readings and Stories of the Early Chinese in Hawaii* (Honolulu, 1975), 101; James G. Y. Ho, "Honolulu Chinatown Fires of 1886–1900–1902," *Downtown Planet*, November 4, 2002, 7.
12. *EBU*, June 16, 1900, 1; John Taksaki, "Kaimuki," HJH, Vol. 9 (1975), 64–74; Charlie Minor [as told to Gail Miyasaki], "Chinatown," in Nancy Foon Young, ed., *Asian-Americans in Hawaii* (Honolulu, 1975), 138–39.

13. Soga, *Gojunenkan No Hawaii Kaiko*, 94; *EBU*, May 7, 1900, 1.

14. Brian Niiya, ed., *Encyclopedia of Japanese History* (New York, 1993), 262; Niiya, *Encyclopedia*, revised edition (New York, 2001), 368; Gary Y. Okihiro, "The Japanese in America," in Niiya, *Encyclopedia*, revised edition, 1–23; Roland Kotani, *Japanese in Hawaii: A Century of Struggle* (Honolulu, 1985); Tom Brislin, *Weep into Silence/Cries of Rage: Bitter Divisions in Hawaii's Japanese Press* (Columbia, S.C., 1995).

15. *HIN*, 422; Chung, *My Seventy-Nine Years in Hawaii*, 196–97; *Star-Bulletin* (Honolulu), February 3, 1999; September 27, 2002.

16. *EBU*, April 18, 1900, 1; Mori File, MAM; Eriko Yamamoto, *The Evolution of an Ethnic Hospital: An Analysis of Ethnic Processes of Japanese Americans in Honolulu through the Development of the Kuakini Medical Center* (Ph.D. diss., University of Hawaii at Manoa, 1988).

17. Day File, MAM.

18. Emerson File, MAM.

19. Wood File, MAM.

20. Hoffman File, MAM.

21. Carmichael File, MAM. On the plague crisis in San Francisco, see Guenter Risse, "'A Long Pull, a Strong Pull, and All Together': San Francisco and Bubonic Plague, 1907–1908," *Bulletin of the History of Medicine*, Vol. 66 (1992), 260–82; Risse, "The Politics of Fear: Bubonic Plague in San Francisco, California, 1900," in Linda Bryder and Derek A. Dow, eds., *New Countries and Old Medicine: Proceedings of an International Conference on the History of Medicine and Health* (Auckland, N.Z., 1995); Risse, "No Burning: Race, Public Health, and Civil Rights in San Francisco's Chinatown, 1900," Policy History Conference, May 31, 2002; Susan Craddock, *City of Plagues: Disease, Poverty, and Deviance in San Francisco* (Minneapolis, 2000); Nayan Shah, *Contagious Divides: Epidemics and Race in San Francisco's Chinatown* (Berkeley, 2001); and Marilyn Chase, *The Barbary Plague: The Black Death in Victorian San Francisco* (New York, 2003).

22. *HIN*, 522, 527–28.

23. Thurston quoted in *PCA*, November 8, 1887, 2. Thurston was using "plague" metaphorically at the time and probably referring to leprosy, but his old fears applied even more forcefully and literally with the arrival of bubonic plague itself; *HIN*, 423–31.

24. *PCA*, March 1, 1900, 3; *IND*, March 7, 1900, 4, March 11, 1900, 5; Katsuki File, MAM. Katsuki eventually decided to remain in Honolulu, where he had a long and successful practice. When he died in 1967 at the age of 101, he was considered the dean of Hawaii's medical community.

25. David Selvin, *Sky Full of Storm: A Brief History of California Labor* (San Francisco, 1975); Robert Edward Wynne, *Reaction to the Chinese in the Pacific Northwest and British Columbia, 1850–1910* (New York, 1978); Risse, "No Burning: Race, Public Health and Civil Rights in San Francisco's Chinatown,

1900," paper presented at the Policy History Conference, St. Louis, Mo., May 31, 2002; Charles McClain, *In Search of Equality: The Chinese Struggle Against Discrimination in Nineteenth-Century America* (Berkeley, 1994); and McClain, "Of Medicine, Race and American Law: The Bubonic Plague Outbreak of 1900," *Law and Social Inquiry*, Vol. 13 (1988), 447–513; Nayan Shah, *Contagious Divides*; Chase, *Barbary Plague*.

26. See, for example, John G. Grace, "Some Observations on the Plague in Hawaii," *New Zealand Medical Journal*, Vol. 1 (1900–01), 166–68; and Herbert P. Williams, "Honolulu's Contention with the Plague," *The Sanitarian* (1900), 319–28.

27. Galbraith File, MAM; *PCA*, January 27, 1900, 9; J. J. Kinyoun to Walter Wyman, December 6, 1900, in *Operations of the United States Marine-Hospital Service, 1901* (Washington, D.C. [1902]), 499.

28. J. J. Kinyoun, "The Prophylaxis of Plague," *Journal of the American Medical Association*, Vol. 42 (1904), 235; "Directions for Combating Plague," forwarded to Washington, D.C., by the U.S. consul-general in Berlin, then reprinted in *United States Public Health Reports*, Vol. 17, Part 2 (1902), 2371–73; Eduardo Liceaga, "The Bubonic Plague" [American Public Health Association, New York], *Public Health Papers and Reports*, Vol. 32, Part 1 (1906), 215–18; Mark Gamsa, "The Epidemic of Pneumonic Plague in Manchuria, 1910–11, in Historiographical Perspective," draft of a paper, kindly provided by the author; Rupert Blue, "The Prophylaxis and Eradication of Plague," *California State Journal of Medicine*, Vol. 5 (1907), 306.

29. Kinyoun, "The Prophylaxis of Plague," 235.

30. *HIN*, 424; D[uncan]. A. Carmichael to Surgeon General, October 15, 1900, in *Annual Report of the Supervising Surgeon-General of the Marine-Hospital Service of the United States for the Fiscal Year 1900* (Washington, D.C. [1901]), 440.

31. On the Philippines, see Ken De Bevoise, *Agents of Apocalypse: Epidemic Disease in the Colonial Philippines* (Princeton, 1995), 177, 181–82, 242, n. 29, and Reynaldo C. Ileto, "Cholera and the Origins of the American Sanitary Order in the Philippines," in David Arnold, ed., *Imperial Medicine and Indigenous Societies* (Manchester and New York, 1988), 125–48. The battle against yellow fever in Panama is the subject of dozens of books.

32. *IND*, April 30, 1900, 1; *Boston Herald*, quoted in *IND*, February 2, 1900, 4.

33. See William Deverell, "Plague in Los Angeles, 1924: Ethnicity and Typicality," in Valerie J. Matsumoto and Blake Allmendinger, eds., *Over the Edge: Remapping the American West* (Berkeley, 1999), 172–200.

34. *PCA*, January 1, 1900, 14.

Index